A Technical Manual for Health Care Providers

Caring for Women with Circumcision

NAHID TOUBIA, MD

with foreword by Donna Shalala

and introduction by Allan Rosenfield

A *RAINBO* PUBLICATION

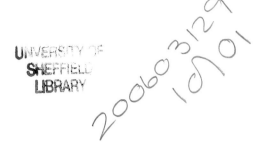

This manual was developed as part of the *Global Action Against Female Genital Mutilation (GAAFGM)* project, a joint effort between RAINBO and the Joseph F. Mailman School of Public Health of Columbia University, New York.

Partial support provided under a cooperative agreement from the Health Resources and Services Administration (HRSA) through the Association of Schools of Public Health (ASPH) and The US Public Health Service Office on Women's Health (PHS OWH)

Support for this project was also provided by the Ford Foundation, Public Welfare Foundation, New York Community Trust and the Open Society Foundation

Published by RAINBO
915 Broadway, Suite 1109, New York, NY 10010
Tel: (212) 477-3318 Fax: (212) 477-4154
Email: rainbq@aol.com
     www.rainbo.org

Edited by: Cynthia J. Laitman, MS, Managing Editor, *Annals of Surgery*
Designed by: Davidson Design, Inc., New York
Printed by: Virginia Lithograph, Arlington, Virginia

Note: The information, views and opinions contained in this book are the sole responsibility of the author.

ISBN 1-893136-0109

Library of Congress Catalog Card Number: 99-61020

CONTENTS

ACKNOWLEDGEMENTS

I would like to thank **Katherine Hall Martinez, J.D.**, Staff Attorney, International Program, the Center for Reproductive Law and Policy (CRLP), New York, who contributed technical legal analysis and advice to chapter 8 and throughout the manual.

Special thanks to **Eileen Coneely**, **Zeinab Eyega**, and **Tagreid Abu-Hassabo** of Research, Action and Information Network for the Bodily Integrity of Women (RAINBQ) for their substantive contribution and effort in overseeing and managing the development and production of this manual.

Many thanks to the following individuals who have generously contributed their time as members of the Advisory Committee to the project, reviewers of several drafts, and as members of the Users Focus Group which undertook post-development testing:

Raqiya D. Abdalla
Former Vice Minister of Health, Somalia
Consultant, Reproductive Health, Anandale, Virginia

Nancy Bolan, RN, MPH, FNP
Family Nurse Practitioner, Brooklyn Hospital Center, Department of Family Practice, Brooklyn, New York

Peter Bernstein, MD, MPH
Assistant Professor, Department of Obstetrics and Gynecology and Women's Health, Albert Einstein College of Medicine, Montefiore Medical Center, Queens, New York

Sylvia Crescencia Chipiro-Mupepi, M Ed (Ad Ed)
Former Interim Deputy Director, Nursing Services, Zimbabwe;
Candidate for Ph.D. Nursing, University of Michigan, Ann Arbor

Nicholas Cunningham, MD, DrPH
Professor of Clinical Pediatrics and Clinical Public Health; Director, Division of General Pediatrics, Columbia University College of Physicians and Surgeons, New York, New York

Beverly Ellis, FNP
Director, Family Nurse Practitioner Program, College of Nursing at SUNY Downstate, Brooklyn, New York

Betty Farrell, CNM, MSN, MPH
Consultant Health Services Training, New York, New York

Mark Gray, MD
Private practice, Obstetrics and Gynecology, New York, New York

Betty Hambleton
Senior Advisor, Women's Health, Health Resources and Services Administration, Bethesda, Maryland

Hilda Hutcherson, MD
Assistant Professor of Obstetrics and Gynecology, Columbia Presbyterian Hospital, New York, New York

Carol Horowitz, MD, MPH
Assistant Professor of Health Policy and Medicine, Mount Sinai Medical Center, New York, New York

Virginia Jackson, RN, MSN, CNM
Consultant, Women's Health , Briarcliff, New York

Timothy Johnson, MD

Professor and Chair, Obstetrics and Gynecology, University of Michigan, Ann Arbor

Wanda K. Jones, DrPH

Deputy Assistant Secretary for Health (Women's Health), U.S. Department of Health and Human Services, Washington, D.C.

Allan S. Keller, MD

Program Director, Bellevue/New York University Program for Survivors of Torture; Assistant professor of Clinical Medicine, New York University School of Medicine; Attending Physician, New York University School of Medicine, New York, New York

Jennifer LaFontant, MD

Chief of Obstetrics and Gynecology, Lincoln Medical Center, New York, New York

Saralyn Mark, MD

Senior Medical Advisor, Department of Health and Human Services, Office on Women's Health, Washington, D.C.

Ahmed Moen, DrPH

Associate Professor and Interim Director of Health Sciences Management; Division of Allied Health Sciences, Howard University, Washington, D.C.

Shrine Mohagheghpour, MSc

Program Specialist, Division of Women's Health Issues, American College of Obstetricians and Gynecologists, Washington, D.C.

Jacques Moritz, MD

Assistant Clinical Professor of Obstetrics and Gynecology, Columbia College of Physicians and Surgeons, New York, New York

Nawal Nour, MD

Obstetrician/Gynecologist, Brigham and Women's Hospital, Boston, Massachusetts

Kowser Omer-Hashi

Former Nurse Midwife, Somalia; Reproductive Health Consultant, Toronto, Canada

Harriet Ozer, BA, MA, BSN, CNM

Midwife, Jacobi Medical Center, Bronx, New York

Pat Paluzzi, CNM, MPH

Associate Medical Director, Planned Parenthood Maryland, Baltimore, Maryland

Janna Rehnstrom, MD

Gynecologist, Lenox Hill Hospital, St. Luke's Roosevelt Hospital, New York, New York

Carolyn M. Sampselle, PhD, RNC

Professor of Nursing, Department of Obstetrics and Gynecology, Medical School & Women's Studies, Literature Science and the Arts, University of Michigan, Ann Arbor

Katherine Sherif, MD

Assistant Professor of Medicine, Medical College of Pennsylvania, Philadelphia

David Smith, PhD

Associate Director, Office of International and Refugee Health, U.S. Department of Health and Human Services, Rockville, Maryland

Jini Tanenhaus

Physician's Assistant, Planned Parenthood New York City, New York, New York

Susan Xenarios, CSW

Director, Crime-Victims Treatment Center, St. Luke's-Roosevelt Hospital, New York, New York

Finally, my deepest gratitude goes to the African women immigrants and refugees who were courageous enough to share their personal experiences on female circumcision and their encounters with the health care systems in host countries. I hope that this book is a step towards facilitating the quality of health care services they deserve.   **N.T.**

FOREWORD

By Donna E. Shalala

Secretary, U.S. Department
of Health and Human Services

This is a manual for health care providers who, for the first time, may be encountering conditions in women that result from female circumcision/female genital mutilation. Female circumcision/female genital mutilation is a term used for a number of different cultural practices involving cutting, removal and sometimes sewing up the external female genitalia. It is practiced widely in certain parts of Africa, as well as in some parts of Southeast Asia. Women who come from these cultures have immigrated to the United States and live throughout the country, although they are concentrated in eight or ten urban areas. Women who have been the victims of these unnecessary genital surgeries often suffer lifelong medical and psychological consequences.

International organizations, as well as many governments of the immigrants' natal countries, have recognized that female circumcision/female genital mutilation is a violation of the human rights of girl children. The World Health Organization has recognized that female circumcision/female genital mutilation causes lasting health problems. Yet the practice continues and some immigrants would continue it here in the United States. The practice is illegal in the United States and my Department is working to let people know this. More importantly, my Department has launched outreach programs to educate mothers, fathers and grandparents about the lasting medical and psychological consequences of these practices.

Many health practitioners in the United States will have never encountered female circumcision/female genital mutilation or its physiological aftermath. Most often they will see a woman who is pregnant or in labor, and will confront medical decisions that must be made quickly and which they have never before considered. For this reason, as well as to help train new health care practitioners, my Department has been pleased to support RAINBQ in producing this manual. It is intended to benefit all women and girls who suffer from the complications of female circumcision/female genital mutilations.

As an African woman and a physician I have long
been aware of the problems, both social and physical, of the practice of
female circumcision (FC). For many years I have been outspoken about
this cruel and unfair tradition in my own country, Sudan, where the
severest form of genital cutting and sewing is the norm. But I have
always known that cruelty is not what motivates parents to subject their
daughters to this socially prescribed requirement. I have also known the
silent, and not so silent, suffering of hundreds of women who presented
to public hospital clinics where I worked or who trusted me with very
painful details of their lives in my private office or after I gave a public
lecture against the practice. But my lips were sealed whenever I lived in
the West; first in England and Wales to acquire my surgical training and
more recently in the United States when I worked for an international
health research organization.

Talking about this issue in the West felt like revealing my family's dys-
functional behavior to their in-laws. I had a mixed sense of shame and
loving protection towards my African heritage that made me want to
resolve the issue internally and not involve our historical adversaries.
Unfortunately, my country and others of the horn of Africa were soon
devastated by civil war and famine. Overnight I found myself a member
of the African community of exiles, refugees and immigrants in the
United States which, by the mid 1990's, have reached a few hundred
thousands. Female circumcision (FC) or female genital mutilation
(FGM), as it is controversially labeled, became a topic of daily coverage
in American media outlets from national newspapers to the smallest
local publication as well as radio and television. Nothing else, whether
positive or negative, that happened in Africa or was brought by Africans
to the U.S. has ever claimed such widespread attention as this issue. The
reason behind that unprecedented attention still escapes me. What I
have come to learn through the years is that this reaction is not unique
to the U.S. and that similar attention, and extreme moral indignation,
have been expressed in Europe and other Western countries where
Africans took refuge in the past two decades.

An understandable measure taken or contemplated by host countries is
to pass laws criminalizing and prohibiting the practice on their soil. It
was always clear to the specialists that passing of specific anti-FGM
laws is not a legal necessity since all Western countries have adequate
child protection and assault laws to prosecute those practicing
FC/FGM. The most glaring evidence is that the only Western country
which ever prosecuted a circumciser or a parent is France, a country
that does not have specific anti-FGM laws. Passing a criminal law, in the
case of FC/FGM, is for the most part a political statement that such

practices will not be tolerated. The publicity generated around the new law is often used to send a strong message to those who may entertain the thought of importing this practice to the new land.

While supporting some of the political and legal actions taken by the host society I was, nonetheless, saddened and angered by the lack of concern for the feelings of the community, and particularly the women. For centuries they were surrounded by the belief that, to circumcise your daughter is the proper and noble thing to do. Then, for reasons usually outside their control, they take a short airplane ride, and they are transported to another culture that sees them as social pariahs, barbaric mutilators or pitifully mutilated individuals. Most of the time they are excluded from discussions that involve their lives and their bodies and they are rarely invited to contribute to the solution. Ultimately, many of them present themselves to health clinics, mostly because of pregnancy and for childbirth. Health care professionals, who are totally unprepared for their needs, may try to do their best but often say or do the wrong things.

In 1993, when Representative Patricia Shroeder and the congressional women's caucus, drafted the bill for an anti-FGM law, a group of African and U.S. physicians and lawyers sent them suggestions for amendments to the proposed legal language and other measures without which passing of a criminal law would become an act of persecution and not promotion of justice. These included suggestions for training health care and social service providers and involving the African community through outreach measures. To their credit, all suggestions were included, and when congress passed the criminal law in 1996, it also passed directives to the Department of Health and Human Services (DHSS) to undertake community education and outreach and to provide training to health personnel. This directive started a rewarding and collegial relationship with several senior employees of the DHHS who gave financial support to this manual and provided technical advise in their personal capacity as professionals.

When we started the organization RAINBQ in 1994, our main objective was to act as the catalyst for the social change needed in Africa that focuses attention on the protection of women's rights and would result in societal rejection of FC/FGM. By 1995 the need for programs to serve the African immigrant community in the U.S. and other host countries became very evident. We heard frequent complaints from circumcised women seeking health care in the U.S. We also believed in our souls that social change will not be attained through legal or punitive action alone, and that one of the best ways to engage mothers in a new way of thinking regarding their daughters is by addressing their own health needs first. In the second half of 1995 and early 1996 the Immigrant Program at RAINBQ undertook a needs-assessment study in New York City. The study surveyed health and social service providers in 11 public hospitals and several maternal and child health clinics. The study also included in-depth interviews with African women and men. Though brief, the study identified many needs expressed by service providers and their clients, which guided us in compiling the present manual.

Meanwhile, staff from the Immigrant Program were conducting reproductive health training and consultations with African refugee and immigrant women. Through interacting with these women, listening to their feelings, opinions, wisdom and experiences we learned much of the client's perspectives and cultural sensibilities that are included in this volume. This process confirmed our long held belief that, by building a relationship of trust, the physician, nurse or social worker can play a crucial role in empowering a circumcised woman to understand what happened to her, overcome her own pain and anger, and stand up to protect her daughter against circumcision. I know that those who helped develop this reference manual hold this expressed belief and they gave generously of their time to this project in the hope that through their contribution they have helped circumcised women as well as contributed to stopping the practice. We invite all those who are engaged in the daily challenges of providing services to these women to join us in this belief and help create a humane example of facilitating social change.

Nahid Toubia
New York, January 1999

AUTHOR'S NOTE

INTRODUCTION

By Allan Rosenfield, MD

Dean, Joseph F. Mailman School of Public Health,
Columbia University

An estimated 130 million girls and women have undergone female circumcision (FC)—also known as female genital mutilation (FGM.) Most of these women and girls live in Africa and some in Asia where in their individual countries the practice is a tradition. However, with the influx of immigration, increasing numbers of these women now live in Europe, the United States, Canada, Australia and New Zealand. In recent years many of these countries have found it necessary to issue laws on FC/FGM to prevent the propagation of the practice.

The debate on FC/FGM has evoked several questions that have yet to be resolved. Some of these questions, for example, concern the right of an individual or a group to preserve their cultural beliefs and practices in a host country. Do people—parents or other members of a group—have the right to alter the body of a child in the name of tradition? Should an adult have the right to choose and consent to non-therapeutic medical or ritualistic altering of their bodies? While the debate on those issues continues, the fact remains that circumcised women and girls in host countries are faced with health care providers who have little if any information on FC/FGM, and who are not trained in the management of its complications. Fortunately, one thing that is not under debate is the right to health and to receiving appropriate healthcare services.

According to the Center for Diseases Control (CDC) an estimated 168,000 girls and women living in the United States in 1990 who came from FC/FGM practicing countries or regions either had or may have been at risk for FC/FGM. The addition of a large number of immigrant women from FC/FGM practicing countries to the map of health care consumers has impacted the health care practice in the U.S. and other host countries. Many physicians and other health care practitioners have expressed their need for training materials that furnish accurate clinical information on the practice. *Caring for Women with Circumcision: A Reference Manual for Health Care Providers* comes in a timely fashion to fill a void and bridge a gap translating policy making and legislation into the clinical stead. It is a technical guide on how to manage the clinical as well as the social aspects of circumcised women within the context of host countries' health services systems. The book provides a thorough overview of FC/FGM-related physical complications and their clinical management, as well as para-natal and obstetric care for circumcised women. The illustrations make a first time clinical encounter with a circumcised woman a more efficient one. The book also provides an illustrated step-by-step guidance through the process of defibulation.

The practice of female circumcision/female genital mutilation is a highly complex issue that ties into traditional gender roles, superstition, local concepts on health and sexuality, as well as several other social relations. In a clinical situation, a health care provider must be equipped to handle a circumcised woman without jeopardizing her health and physical integrity, or subjecting her to unnecessary feelings of humiliation and alienation. If handled inappropriately, circumcised women may find the clinical encounter traumatic, and may thus respond by denying themselves health care thus risking their health and, for pregnant women, that of their fetus. The manual furnishes an informational background for health care providers on the social and cultural meanings of FC/FGM, and serves as a reference in identifying the immigrant communities from FC/FGM practicing cultures, their family structure and other support systems, and their group and individual characteristics. It offers guidelines for culturally sensitive counseling and outreach. Furthermore, the manual has case studies that further prepare the health care provider and provide more insight into the clinical encounter with a circumcised woman.

Since 1994, ten states have passed legislation prohibiting the practice of FC/FGM and instituting criminal sanctions. In 1996 a federal law criminalizing the practice was passed and a congressional mandate was issued for the Department of Health and Human Services (DHHS) to develop materials to train physicians and nurses on how to treat circumcised women. This manual provides an overview of the legal status in the U.S. and legal issues involved in caring for circumcised women, and supplies health care providers with information on reporting to authorities and counseling the patient on the law.

Most international and regional Human Rights Declarations have proclaimed FC/FGM a violation to women's health and rights. Indeed, there is a global effort to address FC/FGM to which families and activists both in FC/FGM practicing countries and abroad, and nongovernmental and governmental organizations contribute. As professionals who participate in the provision of health care services to women I urge you to partake in that expansive effort by delivering the appropriate health care services to circumcised women. This highly informative and professional book is a tool that will help you achieve this goal.

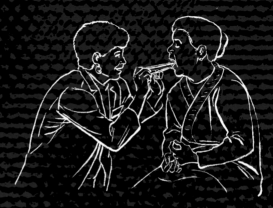

AN INTRODUCTION TO FEMALE CIRCUMCISION/ FEMALE GENITAL MUTILATION

What is FC/FGM?

Female circumcision (FC), or female genital mutilation (FGM) as it is also known, is the collective name given to traditional practices that involve the cutting of female genitals.

In 1995, the World Health Organization (WHO) recommended a standardized typology of FC/FGM which is a broad framework designed to encompass both common and rare procedures. The intent is to emphasize a complete "hands-off" policy towards ritual genital cutting. The preamble for the WHO classification states:

"Female genital mutilation is a deeply rooted, traditional practice. However, it is a form of violence against girls and women that has serious physical and psychosocial consequences which adversely affect health. Furthermore, it is a reflection of discrimination against women and girls.

WHO is committed to the abolition of all forms of female genital mutilation. It affirms the need for the effective protection and promotion of the human rights of girls and women, including their rights to bodily integrity and to the highest standard of physical, mental, and social well being.

WHO strongly condemns the medicalization of female genital mutilation. That is, the involvement of the health professions in any form of female genital mutilation in any setting, including hospitals or other health establishments."

Although articles and study reports published before 1995 may have used different classifications, it is strongly recommended that health care providers and researchers use the standardized WHO classification to establish more effective professional communication and unified criteria for research.

WHO Classification

TYPE I
Excision of the prepuce with or without excision of part or all of the clitoris.

Note: It is not easy to capture this type in a photograph. Type 1 is commonly missed during an examination by an inexperienced clinician.

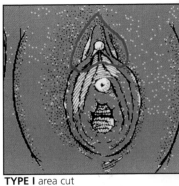

TYPE I area cut

TYPE II
Excision of the prepuce and clitoris together with partial or total excision of the labia minora.

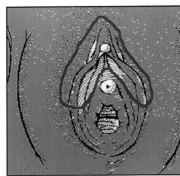

TYPE II area cut

TYPE III
Excision of part or all of the external genitalia and stitching/narrowing of the vaginal opening (infibulation).

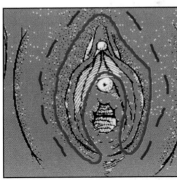

TYPE III area cut

TYPE IV Unclassified

- Pricking, piercing or incision of the clitoris and/or labia

- Stretching of the clitoris and/or labia

- Cauterization by burning of the clitoris and surrounding tissues

- Scraping (angurya cuts) of the vaginal orifice or cutting (gishiri cuts) of the vagina.

- Introduction of corrosive substances into the vagina to cause bleeding or herbs into the vagina with the aim of tightening or narrowing the vagina.

- Any other procedure that falls under the definition of female genital mutilation.

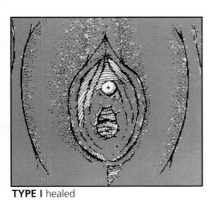

TYPE I healed

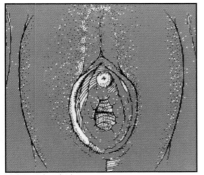

TYPE II healed

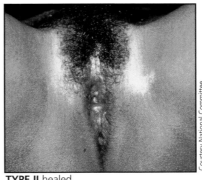

TYPE II healed

Courtesy, National Committee
Against Excision, Burkina Faso

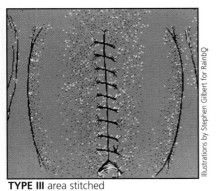

TYPE III area stitched

Illustrations by Stephen Gilbert for RainbØ

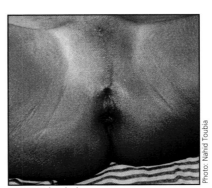

TYPE III healed

Photo: Nahid Toubia

The greatest controversy arises regarding different descriptions of Type I FC/FGM. Many writers describe Type I as removal of the prepuce of the clitoris without the glans, making it analogous to male circumcision. Review of the literature shows that clinicians who actually examine women reported that the overwhelming majority of cases considered to be Type I are, in fact, clitoridectomies; that is the glans or a portion of the body of the clitoris is removed.

While terminology can be precise, the performance of the surgery frequently is not. Conditions under which the procedures occur are usually not conducive to accurate cutting nor are the majority of operators trained medical personnel. Often, those performing the procedure are traditional circumcisers and barbers, or other individuals designated to do this work. The circumciser may have poor eyesight or shaky hands, the lighting may be poor, and the unanesthetized child may be screaming and wriggling. In addition, the instrument of cutting (these can range from a scalpel to a piece of glass) may be dull and cause tearing of the flesh rather than a clean incision.

This means that although the patient may come from a social group known to perform a certain type of circumcision, she may have more (or less) damage than would be expected. For example, some patients from Nigeria who were expected to have Type II FC/FGM, were found on examination to have deeper cuts of the labia that healed by fusion of the wound's edges, resulting in an infibulating type scar.

Conversely, patients who have been infibulated (Type III) and theoretically should have no clitoris at all may, in fact, have a partially or totally intact clitoris under the stitched labia majora. The latter possibility is particularly important to remember when performing defibulation or removal of a cyst. (See Chapters 3 and 4)

Recording Types of FC/FGM

Although the WHO classification is comprehensive, in actual practice the three most commonly encountered types of FC/FGM are:

1 **Clitoridectomy:** in which part or all of the clitoris is removed (Type I.)

2 **Excision:** which involves partial or total removal of the clitoris and labia without stitching (Type II.)

3 **Infibulation:** in this type, the clitoris and labia minora are excised and the incised sides of the labia majora are stitched together, creating a false hood of skin over the urethra and anterior part of the vaginal orifice (Type III.) In West Africa another type of infibulation was found where the labia minora (and not the labia majora) were used to create an infibulation hood of skin over the vulva.

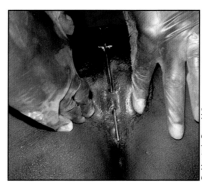

Labia Minora Infibulation

A clinical examination is necessary to establish the type of FC/FGM or the exact degree of cutting. Recording the circumcision type on the basis of the patient's knowledge is not reliable unless it is clearly established that she was informed after a previous examination by a knowledgeable clinician.

WHO is currently working to have the above classification incorporated into the International Classification of Diseases (ICD) coding system. Currently in the U.S. there is no requirement to report cases of FC/FGM in adults or children to the Center for Disease Control (CDC) for statistical purposes. There is no information at present regarding requirements for medical statistical reporting in other countries. Regardless of medical regulatory requirements, accurate recording in the patient's notes is important to facilitate collection of statistics in the future. (For legal requirements of reporting cases in children please see Chapter 5.)

Functional Anatomy of the Female External Genitals

In order to understand the damage caused by FC/FGM and the potential clinical complications that may arise from the cutting and healing process a close look at the functional anatomy and histology of the clitoris, labia minora and majora is necessary. The clitoris is the specialized sexual organ of the girl and although only the highly sensitive glans and part of the shaft is visible externally part of the body and the two crura are embedded behind the symphysis pubis. This means that in most types of FC/FGM a substantial amount of clitoral tissue may still be intact unless the whole clitoris have been dissected out and avulsed from its insertion in the pubic bone.

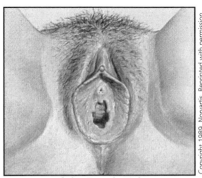

Anatomy of the Female Vulva

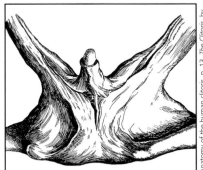

Anatomical Dissection of the Clitoris

Because of the erectile nature of the spongy tissue of the clitoris and the labia minora they both have a high pressure and dense vascular supply that can cause considerable bleeding when cut. The nerve supply is also dense and concentrated making the clitoris and labia highly sensitive to stimulation as well as to pain. The cutting is therefore extremely painful and often results in long term residual pain and discomfort in the area of the scar.

Development of genitals in utero showing the correspondence between male and female genitalia

External genitalia in the ninth week.

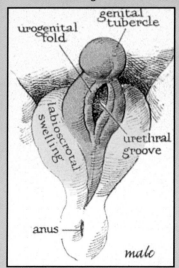
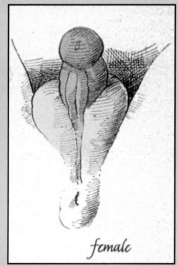

External genitalia in the tenth week.

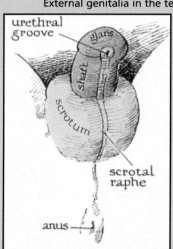
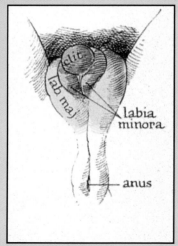

External genitalia at term.

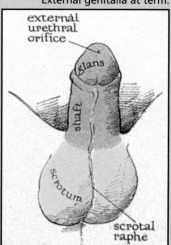
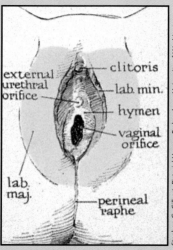

Stephen G. Gilbert. Pictorial Human Embryology, University of Washington Press, 1989, p. 48. "Reprinted with permission of the University of Washington Press"

Review of the anatomy and physiology of the female external genitalia

The term vulva refers to the structures that are visible externally in the perineal region (the area limited anteriorly by the symphysis pubis, posteriorly by the buttocks, and laterally by the thighs).

The mons pubis is a fatty tissue prominence overlying the symphysis. It is covered with coarse, curly pubic hair that forms the escutcheon which appears as a flattened inverted triangle over the symphysis. The appearance of this female escutcheon may vary in some women. The labia majora are two longitudinal folds of adipose tissue extending from the mons to enclose the labia minora and structures in the vestibule (the area containing the urethral and vaginal opening). In nulliparous women, the labia majora are usually closely apposed; in multiparous women they may gape. The mons and the labia majora are well supplied with sweat glands, blood and lymphatic vessels, and nerves. The outer surface of the labia is covered with pubic hair, which may extend out to the thighs in some women. The labia minora are thin firm folds of skin, inside and parallel to the majora. Anteriorly they form the clitoral hood (prepuce) and frenulum, they split to enclose the vestibule. The labia minora contain no hair follicles, are rich in sebaceous glands, and are well endowed with blood vessels and nerves, functioning as erectile tissue during sexual intercourse. In some women the minora are hidden by the labia majora; in others, they may protrude somewhat. Although they are paired structures, they may not be symmetrical in appearance.

The clitoris is a small, cylindrical erectile organ. The internal structure consists of two crura covered by fibrous tissue and attached to the inferior pubic ramus. These crura converge to form the clitoral body, which contains the corpora cavernosa, that consists of two erectile structures. The body extends downward beneath the prepuce, ending in the glans. The glans, visible externally, lies between the prepuce and the frenulum. The clitoris is supplied by a branch of the pudendal nerve and is richly supplied with sensory nerve endings responsive to varying types of mechanical and psychoemotional stimuli.

The vestibule lies between the clitoris and the fourchette, which is a slightly raised ridge of tissue marking the posterior joining of the labia; the vestibule is bounded by the labia minora. Within the vestibule are the urethral meatus; the orifices of the Skene's or paraurethral gland on either side of the urethral opening; the orifices of the Bartholin's glands that are found at five and seven o'clock between the hymen and the labia minora; the hymen, a thin membranous fold of tissue over the vaginal opening; and the vaginal opening itself. In parous or sexually active women, the hymen may exist only as small tags of skin. The fossa navicularis, usually obliterated by childbirth, is found between the vaginal opening and the fourchette. Just beneath the vestibule are the vestibular bulbs, highly vascular tissue that becomes congested during sexual excitement.

From "Anatomy and Physiology of the Female Reproductive System" by Patricia Aikins Murphy in "Gynecology Well-Woman Care" by Ronnie Lichtman and Susan Papera, Ed. Appleton and Lange 1990.

AN INTRODUCTION TO FC/FGM

CHAPTER 1

Terminology

One of the most controversial issues is whether to use female circumcision or female genital mutilation as the terminology to describe this group of procedures. Those who promote the use of FGM are concerned with the parallels that may be drawn between male and female circumcision, itself, a highly controversial area of debate. Conversely, proponents of the term female circumcision are sensitive to the fact that the term "female genital mutilation" is often offensive to the circumcised women who do not think of themselves as mutilated or of their families as mutilators. They also voice a concern that mutilation terminology is often used as a means to insult the people and the cultures from which they come.

Historically, the term female circumcision (FC) was used in the international literature until the early 1980s when the term female genital mutilation (FGM) was introduced and became more widely used. In the late 1990s, some writers began using other terms such as female genital surgeries (FGS) and female genital cutting (FGC).

The author of this manual believes that the intent is circumcision and the effect is mutilation; that FGM is currently the term used by many official bodies including the U.N., but that more appropriate terms should be used in the clinical setting where the comfort and well being of the patient must be given highest priority. In consideration of all these concerns, the initials FC/FGM are used in the text when referring to any form of ritual genital cutting in girls and women and a list of terms used in local languages is included in the appendix. (For a further discussion on terminology to use in the clinical encounter, please see chapter 6.)

PREVALENCE AND SOCIO-CULTURAL CHARACTERISTICS

Why is FC/FGM performed?

Female genital cutting in its ritualistic form is done for a variety of reasons. Some societies consider it a rite of passage into womanhood, as in Kenya and Sierra Leone. Others use it as a means of preserving a girl's virginity until marriage, as in Sudan, Egypt, and Somalia. In each community where it is practiced, FC/FGM is considered an important part of the culturally defined gender identity, which explains why many mothers and grandmothers identify with and defend the practice. They consider it a fundamental part of their own womanhood and believe that it is essential to ensuring their daughters' acceptance into their society. In most poor societies, few economic opportunities exist for women outside of marriage; to be circumcised is often a prerequisite for qualifying for wifehood and therefore a critical factor in ensuring social and economic survival for young women.

In summary FC/FGM has complex economic, moral, aesthetic and gender identity reasons for its occurrence. Those of us who would like to see these practices disappear must attend to the complexity of the reasons and realities of those who favor it before we can dialogue with them.

Who performs FC/FGM?

FC/FGM is practiced primarily in 28 countries in Africa across the center of sub-Saharan Africa from Sudan and Somalia in the east, to most of the countries of West Africa. It is also concentrated along the Nile valley from Egypt in the north to Ethiopia, Uganda and Kenya in the south. It is not known in other Arab speaking North African countries, namely, Tunisia, Algeria, Morocco, and Libya, nor in Southern Africa such as South Africa, Namibia, Zambia and Zimbabwe. (See map on page 24.)

In Asia cases have been reported among rural Kurdish women who live in Northern Iraq and among some tribes in other Arab countries neighboring the Horn of Africa such as Oman, southern Saudi Arabia and Yemen. In India the practice is documented among a religious minority, the Daodi Bohra Muslims of Bombay who have communities in India, East Africa and the United States. Information on female circumcision among these communities is sparse and prevalence rates are unknown. Some writers list Pakistan, Indonesia or Malaysia as countries where FC/FGM is practiced, but there is no documented evidence of a widespread use of the practice in these countries.

The custom cuts across religions and is practiced by some Muslims, Christians, and by the Ethiopian Jews (the Falasha, now living in Israel), as well as by followers of traditional African religions.

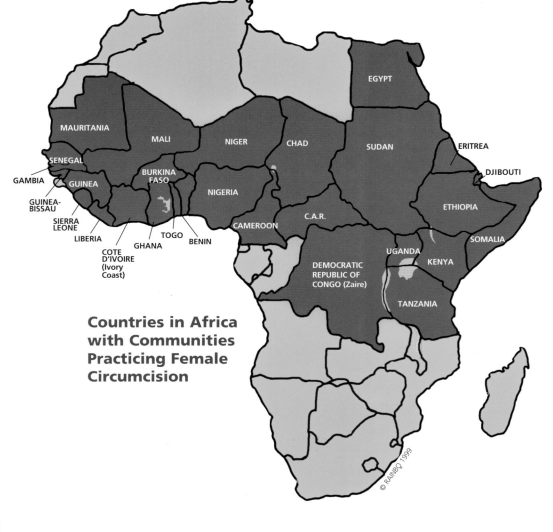

Countries in Africa with Communities Practicing Female Circumcision

Map labels: EGYPT, MAURITANIA, MALI, NIGER, CHAD, SUDAN, ERITREA, DJIBOUTI, SENEGAL, GAMBIA, GUINEA, BURKINA FASO, NIGERIA, ETHIOPIA, GUINEA-BISSAU, C.A.R., CAMEROON, SOMALIA, SIERRA LEONE, TOGO, BENIN, UGANDA, KENYA, LIBERIA, GHANA, COTE D'IVOIRE (Ivory Coast), DEMOCRATIC REPUBLIC OF CONGO (Zaire), TANZANIA

© RAINBO 1999

The chart on page 25 provides an overview of the prevalence rate of FC/FGM by country. Prevalence by country reflects politically defined national boundaries within which the majority or only a few tribes may know the practice. In reality FC/FGM prevails and spreads by ethnic, cultural and religious affiliation of neighboring tribes who may live in different countries. It also lists the most common types in each country. Notice that the prevalence by type can vary dramatically from almost 100% of Type III in Somalia to less than 5% of Type I or II in Uganda.

The physical health effects are more pronounced with infibulation and women with this condition need more attention from the health care system. However it is important to remember that this severe form of FC/FGM constitutes only about 20% of all affected women and is most likely to be seen in women from Somalia, Northern Sudan and Djibouti.

Prevalence Rates and Types of FC/FGM by Country

Prevalence	Country	Type(s) Most Commonly Practiced
50%	**Benin**	Type II
70%	**Burkina Faso**	Type II
20%	**Cameroon**	Types I and II
43%	**Central African Republic**	Types I and II
60%	**Chad**	Type II *[Type III only in eastern parts of the country bordering Sudan]*
5%	**Democratic Republic of Congo (formerly Zaire)**	Type II
43%	**Cote d'Ivoire (Ivory Coast)**	Type II
98%	**Djibouti**	Types II and III
97%	**Egypt**	Types II (72%), I (17%), and III (9%)
95%	**Eritrea**	Types I (64%), III (34%) and II (4%)
90%	**Ethiopia**	Types I and II *[Type III is practiced only in regions bordering Sudan and Somalia]*
80%	**Gambia**	Type II *[Type I practiced only in some parts]*
30%	**Ghana**	Type II
50%	**Guinea**	Type II
50%	**Guinea Bissau**	Types I and II
50%	**Kenya**	Types I and II *[Type III practiced in eastern regions bordering Somalia]*
60%	**Liberia**	Type II
94%	**Mali**	Types I (52%) and II (47%) *[Type III practiced in the southern part of the country (1%)]*
25%	**Mauritania**	Types I and II
20%	**Niger**	Type II
60%	**Nigeria**	Types I and II *[II is predominant in the South and Type III practiced only in the North]*
20%	**Senegal**	Type II
90%	**Sierra Leone**	Type II
98%	**Somalia**	Type III
89%	**Sudan-North**	Types III (82%), I (15%) and II (3%)
18%	**Tanzania**	Types II and III
50%	**Togo**	Type II
5%	**Uganda**	Types I and II

Sources:

Carr D. *Female Genital Cutting: Findings from Demographic and Health Surveys.* Macro International Inc., Sept. 1997.

Office of Asylum Affairs. Bureau of Democracy, Human Rights & Labor. United States Department of State. Washington, D.C. January 1997. *Fact Sheet on Female Genital Mutilation in 16 African Countries: Benin, Burkina Faso, Cote d'Ivoire, Chad, Djibouti, Egypt, Ethiopia, The Gambia, Ghana, Liberia, Mali, Nigeria, Sierra Leone, Somalia, Sudan, Togo.*

Toubia N. *Female Genital Mutilation: A Call for Global Action.* Women, Ink., New York, 1995.

PREVALENCE AND SOCIOCULTURAL CHARACTERISTICS

CHAPTER 2

African Immigrants Statistics in the U.S. and other Western Countries

In the past, the majority of Africans migrating to the West were students who came to further their education; overwhelmingly they were male. Recently, men have brought their wives and families, and younger, more educated women are beginning to arrive as students and professionals. Almost half of all new immigrants from Africa now are women and girls. In addition, thousands of refugee families are being resettled. These immigrants and refugees represent a wide range of social and economic backgrounds, and they have established social support systems and networks in the West that reflect the social and cultural diversity of Africa.

As African immigration increased, circumcised women have come in larger numbers to North America, Western Europe, Australia and New Zealand. Accurate numbers of affected girls and women in these countries are difficult to come by. The International Center for Reproductive Health of the University of Gent, Belgium, conducted a study on FC/FGM among African Immigrants in Europe as part of what is termed the DAPHNE program of the European Commission. The final estimate of that study was still under analysis at the time of publication. In Australia, the Department of Human Services drawing on the figures produced by the Australian Bureau of Statistics Census estimates that 87,000 women and girls from FC/FGM practicing countries lived in that country in 1991.

African immigration to the U.S. has nearly tripled in the past three decades, to almost 25,000 per year in the 1990s. The Centers for Disease Control (CDC) in Atlanta used the 1990 Census data and estimated that approximately 168,000 women and girls who reported ancestry or birth in FC/FGM-practicing countries were in the U.S. and about one fourth of them were under 18 years of age.

Although it is important that these statistical estimates have been generated in the past few years, what is still missing is more studies and documentation of the experiences of African immigrant women in the West and how their physical health, psychological, emotional and social needs may manifest themselves in the new cultural environment. In the following sections, we will reflect on some of the characteristics of the African born population in the U.S., highlight their social systems and the importance of ethnic identity, family, and religion in women's life.

Characteristics of the Population

Although each woman who walks into the clinic is an individual in her own right, it is useful to reflect on some general characteristics that may be common to the cultural groups that practice FC/FGM or may have shaped the individual woman's experience.

Ethnic and national affiliation

Although African immigrants vary in their customs, most have a strong and valued sense of ethnic and national affiliation. Such connections maintain not only one's culture, but also provide financial and moral support. In times of stress, it is the community networks that assist the family, whether through emotional support or collections of money. Health care providers should bear in mind that if these individuals lose their community support system, they may have no one else to turn to. This same community support groups can also assist in mediating between communities and health care, legal and social systems and can often provide valuable translation and mediation services.

Family structures and other systems of support

The family is the most important and influential social institution in almost all African countries, reinforcing and passing on cultural norms from one generation to the next. For many, family obligations and expectations are unaltered by the geographic location of an individual. Among African immigrant and refugee communities, the extended family is commonly involved in decisions that may affect an individual's health care.

Traditional values and methods of relating to each other in many African cultures are hierarchical, and therefore favor respect for authority figures and elders. This hierarchy is reinforced through language, with prescribed terms of address for each person, depending on their status, and who is addressing them. Because of this social power hierarchy some African women may not question the authority of a health care provider. Therefore, if she does not understand or is not satisfied with the services given, she may believe it disrespectful to say so, yet she may not return to the clinic again.

Similar hierarchical systems are common in the relationships between husbands and wives. Women generally fit within a prescribed gender role, where they are the bearers and preservers of culture and the foundation upon which a family survives, while men are the ultimate decision-makers. However, upon immigration to the new society, this hierarchy frequently gets upset. Traditional roles may change as some women take on new responsibilities or work outside the home.

Refugee or Immigrant experience

African refugees and immigrants share the same problems of resettlement common to all immigrants and refugees. When an African immigrant woman visits your practice remember that her main current concern will most likely revolve around issues of cultural adaptation, immigration status, economic hardship and isolation rather than the circumcision that happened many years ago.

The length of time an immigrant or refugee has been in the new country will usually impact on her health care-seeking behaviors and beliefs. Patients who are more recent arrivals may need more explanation of treatments as well as assistance negotiating the system.

A woman's immigration status will also affect her decisions to seek care. With changes in immigration and welfare laws in the U.S., many immigrant women do not have easy access to care when their documents are not in order.

Largest African-Born Populations in the U.S.

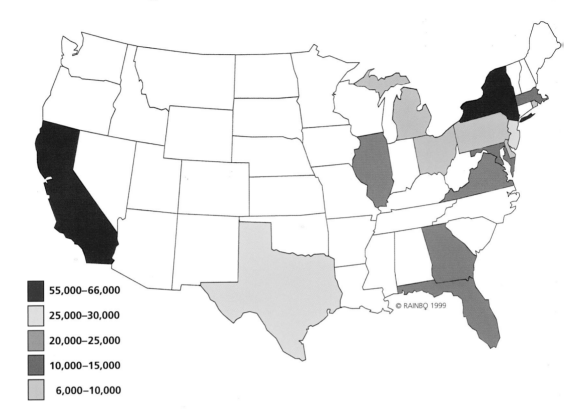

■	55,000–66,000
▫	25,000–30,000
▨	20,000–25,000
▨	10,000–15,000
▨	6,000–10,000

© RAINBO 1999

Education

A woman's level of education is probably one of the most important factors contributing to her health beliefs and health-seeking behavior. In general, an educated woman tends to adhere less to traditional practices and is less likely to defer decision-making to other family members. Her increased access to information often influences her knowledge of her body, her understanding of sexual issues and her requests for clinical management. For example, women with higher education and income tend to request defibulation and so called "re-constructive surgery" more frequently than women with lower education and fewer financial means. The former may also be more inclined to request or accept counseling to deal with emerging emotional issues than the latter.

Age

Age is related to education insofar as younger emigres to the U.S. will have more education than older women, and will be exposed to more information and ideas at a more impressionable time in their lives. An immigrant woman who arrives to the new country in her thirties or forties and who has been married for many years, may be more clear about her cultural identity and more adjusted to being circumcised in comparison to a young girl or a teenager who is transplanted to a new country and is trying hard to adapt, juggling her identity between two cultures. Both will differ from a very young child who was circumcised before she came to her new home and will grow up as an American, Australian or European.

Economic status

African women come from diverse economic backgrounds. While middle and high-income immigrants and professionals may use private physicians, many of those seen in public services are low-income and therefore have little access to services. The latter are less likely to have knowledge of English or employment outside the home. As her health care provider, you may be the woman's only contact with the larger society and therefore a key source of information and referral.

Specific characteristics

Because of regional, ethnic, religious and family differences, it is almost impossible to identify, by her general characteristics, whether a woman is circumcised or approves of the custom or even has heard of it. For example, Southern Sudanese do not traditionally practice FC/FGM and the majority would not have heard of the practice even though the prevalence in Northern Sudan is almost 90%. In assessing the health needs of African women emigres, each girl or woman must be considered individually.

Circumcision experience

Based on anecdotal reports, the impact of circumcision on a woman's psychological and emotional well being, perception of body and self, and sexual experiences vary widely depending on many factors. These factors include the age at the time of circumcision, the circumstances surrounding the event, the type or severity of the procedure, and occurrence of complications.

Sexual experience

As with all women, a circumcised woman's sexual experience and relationship with her partner will influence her perception of her body and her own sexuality. If she has experienced sex with a caring partner within the context of a loving relationship, she will adjust to her circumcision differently from a woman who was rejected by her partner or blamed for the failure of the relationship because she is circumcised. This dynamic can occur irrespective of whether either woman has experienced sexual climax. (For more information on the psychological and sexual experience of circumcised women see section 3.)

Previous contact with the health care system

Rural African women who come to a clinic or a hospital may not have used Western health care in their country of origin, whether because of limited economic means or because no such services were available to them. Women from urban settings are usually familiar with Western style health systems. If a woman's first interaction with modern health care happens to be your clinic, her perception of how she was treated will often determine her acceptance of the treatment prescribed and her decision to seek subsequent care.

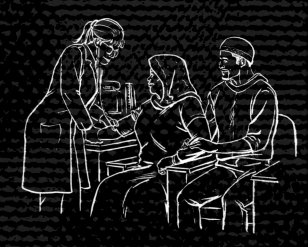

Chapter 3 MEDICAL AND GYNECOLOGICAL CARE

Health Complications of FC/FGM

In the local context within which most FC/FGM traditionally occurs several short- and long-term complications have been reported. Most short-term complications occur because of unsanitary operating conditions, botched procedures by inexperienced circumcisers or inadequate medical services once a complication occurs. In the short term, profuse bleeding is common due to cutting of the high-pressure clitoral vessels. Shock can also occur from loss of blood combined with extreme pain when the procedure is performed without anesthesia. These conditions have sometimes been fatal. Infection of varying degrees from superficial wound infection to septicaemia is also common. Urinary retention from pain and inflammation as well as direct obstruction (in Type III) often occurs in the first few days.

For a full review of documented complications see *Female Genital Mutilation: An Overview* by Nahid Toubia and Susan Izett published by the World Health Organization.

Amongst immigrant clients physicians will rarely encounter short-term complications since FC/FGM is illegal in host countries including the U.S. where girls will hopefully not be circumcised at all. In some cases girls will be circumcised in another country, or, if circumcised locally, are unlikely to be brought to health care facilities for treatment of complications for fear of legal repercussions. Clinicians in host countries are far more likely to encounter the long-term consequences of the procedure such as partial blockage of the urinary meatus, sebaceous and inclusion dermoid cysts, keloid scars, and reproductive tract infections.

In addition to physical complications, a host of sexual and psychological issues will undoubtedly emerge over time as more women become aware of what was done to them, and begin to talk about their personal experiences. Little has been reported in the professional literature about how to handle these particular counseling needs. Overall, the full extent of long-term complications from FC/FGM, including range and prevalence, has yet to be documented.

Most protocols for treatment of FC/FGM complications emphasize the physical problems of infibulation even though that form of FC/FGM constitutes only 20% of all circumcised women. Few published papers and treatment protocols attempt to deal with the physical problems that may result from the less severe types or with the complex psychological, sexual and relationship issues that may occur with any type, and how the physical and mental are not always easy to separate. The following is an attempt to fill in the gaps with the experience of the author, reviewers and other contributors but much more work is needed before appropriate services are provided for circumcised girls and women.

Clinical Presentations and Management

While the clinician in the United States and other Western settings may occasionally have women patients whose presenting complaint involves symptoms and signs of FC/FGM complications, it is more likely that he or she will encounter circumcised women with symptoms not directly attributed to their circumcision.

Many women who have been circumcised may experience gynecological complications and seek treatment for them, but may be reluctant to openly acknowledge problems or issues related to their circumcision. In addition, some women may not show their symptoms until they are advanced and cannot be hidden because they are unaccustomed to seeking medical care because of poor availability of care in their home countries.

A sensitive gynecological and sexual history should be elicited on the first and subsequent visits. Many women may have a sense of physical modesty for having symptoms related to their genitals and may not want to reveal them to strangers. Others may have superstitious beliefs as to what is happening to them, such as growing penises, or have a fear of cancer that they want to hide or deny. They should be welcomed by the provider, and the opportunity should be taken to advise them on the importance of prevention and early treatment.

I External Signs and Symptoms

Complications may be visible and directly related to the circumcision such as:

Ulcer

Vulvar ulcers under the hood of skin of infibulated women have been reported. The condition may be caused by urea crystals precipitated from urine trapped under the hood, forming small stones.

Management

Opening of part or all of the infibulation hood (defibulation) may be necessary to improve drainage. A woman's consent must be obtained after explaining the pathology and the reason for the procedure. The opportunity should be taken to counsel her against re-infibulation. The ulcer may then heal on its own or with topical application of an antibiotic with or without 1% hydrocortisone cream. If the ulcer is chronic it may need excision of the tough fibrous walls before it can heal.

General tenderness and sensitivity in vulva, perineum or vagina

Excessive scarring of the vulva and perineum may cause chronic tenderness and general sensitivity. Some patients reported severe dyspareunia which interfered with sexual intercourse. The psychological and physical contributors to these conditions may never be ascertained and the treatment should be reassurance and soothing treatments such as warm salt baths (sitz baths). Referral for psycho-therapeutic counseling may be considered by the health care provider, where techniques such as behavior modification, desensitization or dilatation may prove useful.

Sebaceous and inclusion (dermoid) cysts

Cysts resulting from embedding of a skin fold in the scar or a sebaceous cyst from the blockage of the sebaceous gland duct are one of the most common complications of all types of FC/FGM. A woman may present

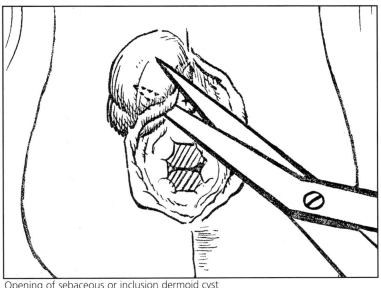

Opening of sebaceous or inclusion dermoid cyst

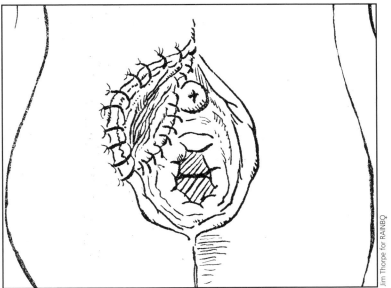

Marsupialization of cyst by stitching it edges to vulval mucosa

with these early on when they are the size of a pea or after they have grown to the size of a tennis ball or a grapefruit.

Management

Small and non-infected cysts may be left alone or removed under local or regional anaesthesia. The most important consideration when deciding whether to interfere with a small cyst is to question if the procedure could result in further damage and scarring of existing sensitive tissue. If such a risk presents itself the woman should be fully informed and her choice on whether to proceed with removal must be with full understanding of that risk.

Large or infected cysts must be excised or marsupialized, usually under general anaesthesia, taking extreme care not to further damage the sensitive tissue or to injure the blood or nerve supply of the area.

Keloid

Many circumcised women have dark skin which is known for its increased tendency to form keloidal scar growth.

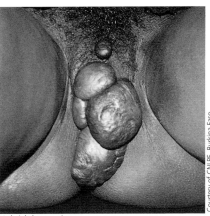

Courtesy of CNLPE, Burkina Faso

Keloidal scar tissue

Management

Keloidal scars are extremely difficult to eliminate since simple excision often results in the growth of more keloidal scar tissue stimulated by the trauma of the cutting. Specialized treatment, usually available in cosmetic surgery units, includes surgical excision followed by application of topical steroids or radiation to suppress the scar reaction. If the keloid scar is minimal, the woman is best advised to leave it undisturbed, and you can reassure her that it has no harmful effects. However, if the scar is large enough to cause difficulties during intercourse, or possible obstruction during delivery, she may be referred to a specialist experienced in removing keloid scars. Some women may be excessively distressed by the presence or appearance of a keloid, and you may consider referring them for surgery for psychological reasons.

Neuroma

The clitoral nerve may get trapped in the fibrous tissue of the scar following clitoridectomy. This may result in an extremely sharp pain over the fibrous swelling anteriorly. The pain may be aggravated by the rubbing of underwear or during intercourse. The neuroma will not be visible but can be diagnosed by testing around the area of the clitoral scar with a delicate object. Under anaesthesia the neuroma may be felt as a small pebble under the mucosa.

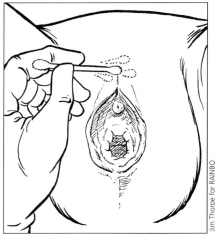

Jim Thorpe for RAINBQ

Clinical testing for area of sensitivity of a neuroma.

Management

There is no reported experience of treatment of this condition. Symptomatic treatment by wearing loose underwear and use of topical Lidocaine cream may be helpful. If the symptoms are severe, surgical excision of the neuroma may be attempted and the nerve end covered with a padding of surrounding mucosa. Before attempting surgery it is important to consider the possibility that the symptoms may have a psychological component as a result of the trauma of the circumcision or from fear of sexual intercourse. The patient may be given therapeutic counseling before and after surgery with this possibility in mind.

Incontinence

Stress incontinence may be due to injury of the external urethral meatus. Less likely to present to a Western clinic is urinary incontinence due to vesico vaginal fistulae (VVF) or fecal incontinence due to vesico-rectal fistula (VRF). VVF and VRF result from prolonged obstructed labor which may occur in some neglected cases of infibulation where a defibulation was not performed.

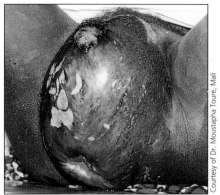

Courtesy of Dr. Moustapha Toure, Mali

Case of obstructed labor resulting in fetal death and both VVF and VRF three days after the onset of labor.

Management

Stress incontinence may be treated with a regimen of pelvic muscle strengthening exercise or referral to a specialized urology unit for repair. Repair of VVF and VRF is a highly specialized and precarious procedure known by only a few surgeons in specialized centers. Full investigation of the centers with good results is advised before the patient is referred.

Vaginal obstruction

Almost complete or semi-complete obstruction of the vaginal outlet in infibulated women or vaginal stenosis from injury or a stone may present with paravaginal hematoma or hematocolpus due to accumulation of menstrual flow. Cases of unmarried girls suspected to be pregnant because of amenorrhea coupled with abdominal swelling have been reported and diagnosed as advanced hematocolpus.

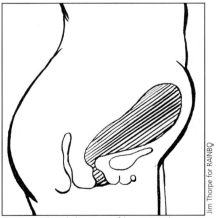

Jim Thorpe for RAINBQ

Cross-sectional diagram of hematocolpus

Management

Surgical incision of an obstructing hood is necessary when the cause is infibulation. In the case of internal vaginal stenosis either mechanical or surgical dilation may be necessary depending on the tightness of the stenosis and the elasticity of the fibrous tissue in the scar.

II Internal Signs and Symptoms

Circumcised women may present with internal symptoms which may or may not be related to their circumcision. These include:

Infections

When circumcised women present with symptoms of urinary tract or pelvic infections, the cause may be related to their circumcision. Urinanalysis and vaginal swabs should be taken to establish the presence and nature of infection. Careful inspection of the vulva will help establish any contributing cause such as an obstruction of urine or vaginal excretions by the hood of skin in infibulated women, the presence of a stricture from a previous injury, or the presence of urinary or vulval stones. Whatever the contributing cause, the obstruction needs to be removed, followed by antibiotic treatment based on the results of the culture and sensitivity test.

Urinary and vaginal stones

Although commonly complicated by infection, urinary and vaginal stones may be the primary presentation. Their causes are the same as those mentioned under infection. They are usually simple to remove but the cause of their occurrence must be dealt with in order to avoid recurrence.

Menstrual disorders

A high percentage of circumcised women report severe or intolerable dysmenorrhea with or without menstrual irregularity. It is not clear if there is a difference in the prevalence or severity of these disorders among circumcised women compared to uncircumcised women since such a controlled study has not been reported. Possible causes of menstrual disorders include an increase in pelvic congestion due to infection, pain or other unknown causes, or worry over the state of the genitals, sexuality or fertility.

Management

Management is the same for circumcised as for uncircumcised women. Counseling to uncover and address worries and anxieties may also be helpful. There is no evidence that any surgical procedure would assist in relieving these symptoms and any such experimentation must be backed by adequate scientific scrutiny.

Referred or systemic symptoms

In countries where the majority of women are circumcised, patients attending gynecological clinics often present with general complaints of dull pelvic and lower back pain, headache and malaise. Physical examination usually reveals no specific or detectable cause for these symptoms. In fact, experience has shown that if this set of symptoms are considered as a general signal from the woman that all is not well, further probing reveals underlying worries regarding her genitals, fertility or problems in her marriage. It is possible that she herself may not be fully aware of her underlying worries and may be projecting them on a somatic cause. Alternatively, she may be partially aware of them and because of shyness or inability to express herself she expects the doctor or nurse to find out what is wrong.

Management

If talking to the patient reveals specific worries such as infertility, treatment may be directed accordingly. If after further probing, including taking a thorough sexual history, the clinician is still unable to identify a particular reason for her symptoms or worries, it is advisable that the patient be referred to a specialized counselor where more time can be devoted to unraveling the cause of the problem.

III No Presenting Symptoms

In many cases the clinician will discover during an examination for an unrelated medical or surgical problem that a woman is circumcised.

Catheterization

A common cause for revealing the circumcision is the need to pass a catheter or attach a urinary bag to monitor urinary output in an unconscious patient or one who is undergoing surgery. Only if the catheterization is impeded by a circumcision scar or a skin hood is special attention necessary and in that case consent from the patient or her guardian is necessary if defibulation is to be performed.

Accidental revealing of circumcision

When circumcision is revealed accidentally while managing an unrelated health aspect, it is sufficient for the health care provider to acknowledge the fact casually and discreetly in a tone that would encourage the woman to ask questions or seek help regarding her circumcision in the future if needed. Otherwise the matter should be dropped and not be made into an issue. (See chapter 6 for a further exploration on how and when to talk about circumcision.)

IV Fertility Concerns

A possible presentation for women with circumcision, particularly those who have suffered from infection, is primary or secondary infertility. Rare cases are documented where the primary cause of infertility was failure of penetration due to a very tight vaginal opening. Treatment constitutes surgical defibulation coupled with sexual counseling for the couple if necessary.

A much more common problem is primary or secondary infertility in a sexually active couple. The differential diagnosis and search for the cause must be approached with the understanding that the infertility may or may not be related to the circumcision. The routine protocol of investigating male causes first should be applied even if the couple shows resistance. In many cultures where FC/FGM is prevalent, fertility is considered a woman's responsibility and the idea that cause or "fault" may be with the man may sometimes be difficult to accept. Professional persuasion may be necessary by educating the patient and her husband about the physiology of conception.

What complicates the issue further is that admitting infertility is still considered shameful in almost all cultures (including the United States and other Western countries) and more so by circumcised women whose society values them by their ability to reproduce. For example, women have been known to come to the clinic complaining of vague and general symptoms hoping that the doctor will find out about their infertility and cure it without the need to admit it.

Finally, circumcised women may need special counseling regarding birth control and family planning depending on the type of circumcision that the woman has, and her contraceptive needs. Certain methods may not be practical for some women, and care should be taken to explain the various options to her and her partner.

V Request for Surgical Correction

Recently, there have been reports of women requesting "re-constructive surgery" of their genitals or some form of reversal of what has been done to them. Most of these requests have come from educated young women who have grown to value their right to bodily integrity.

For infibulated women, a simple defibulation under local or general anaesthesia may be suggested as long as the limitations of the procedure are fully explained. There is a chance that intact sensitive clitoral and labial tissue may lie buried under the infibulation hood and their exposure could enhance sexual feeling in the area. However, such a possibility is not common and cannot be guaranteed. Nevertheless, the surgeon should take extra precautions not to damage any sensitive tissue during the procedure. Examination of the area under the hood—with a good source of light after application of anaesthesia and before cutting—is recommended.

If defibulation is performed for the purposes of enhancing sexual feeling or to overcome sexual problems, it is strongly advised that it should be accompanied by pre- and postoperative sexual counseling with the patient or the couple. This would help bring their expectations in line with what is realistically achievable by surgery, and would explain to them other obstacles to sexual enjoyment and means to overcome them.

There are reports of plastic and urological surgeons suggesting the possibility of successful "re-constructive surgery." While the desire of some women for such a procedure is totally understandable, it is important not to be driven by their need into questionable medical experiments. Reconstruction of a clitoral shaft using erectile tissue from the body of the clitoris usually buried under the mons pubis has been suggested using techniques similar to those used in sex change operations. However, sex change operations are known to have low levels of success, in terms of sexual function. The patient may endure this outcome as a part of the price for achieving the desired change in sex and gender. This is not the case for the FC/FGM patient. Enhanced sexual feeling is probably the most desired and expected outcome; failure to deliver adequate results may lead to extremely dissatisfied and often litigious clients.

This and other issues that are technical or ethical in nature will emerge as more circumcised women access the health care system. The regulating bodies of the medical and nursing professions must monitor and evaluate these issues as they arise.

VI Sexual and Relationship Problems

Those working closely with circumcised women may notice that sexual, marital and relationship problems may be a regular occurrence among this group. Yet most immigrant women do not feel comfortable discussing their private problems with health care providers or social workers who they fear may not understand their culture. As cultures inevitably mix and as younger generations of circumcised women become part of the new society, more may come to their health care providers with their emotional problems. In the absence of studies, it is not possible to compile even a tentative list of the possible sexual or psychological issues or how often they may arise.

It is important that physicians, nurses, social workers, counselors and therapists start with the premise that most, if not all, circumcised women can have a satisfactory sexual and emotional relationship regardless of the degree of their circumcision. The reason for this affirmation is multi-fold. First there is physical evidence. Available scientific data confirm that a substantial percentage of women who have any of the three circumcision types report that they have experienced orgasm at some time. This information is confirmed by intensive interviews with women who have the severest form of infibulation and are informed enough to identify what an orgasm is. They qualified this information by the fact that they were not always sexually satisfied and it was the nature of the relationship and the sensitivity of the partner that made the difference. Second, there are the emotional, sensual, psychological and social aspects to a partnership and a marriage that underlie the sexual. Many couples can have a fulfilling relationship because of the deep emotional bond, camaraderie and social compatibility even if the sexual aspect is not always successful in the clinical sense.

It is possible that with the right partner and, if necessary, the guidance of a sensitive and experienced counselor, most couples can learn to have a fulfilling sexual life.

Chapter 4

OBSTETRICAL CARE OF CIRCUMCISED WOMEN

Pre-natal Care

In a 1996–97 survey of New York City public hospitals, the most common reason for circumcised women to have attended a clinic was for pre-natal care and delivery. Similar results were found in studies conducted in Europe and Australia.

A woman seeking prenatal care may present with any of the three common types of FC/FGM. Her circumcision may be revealed during history taking or during the physical examination. The health care provider must communicate with her that he or she acknowledges the patient's circumcision and is comfortable with the situation and will not over- react or pretend it does not exist. This simple exchange will put the patient at ease and create a basis for a trusting patient-doctor or patient-nurse relationship.

Once this preliminary communication is accomplished, the clinician must determine if the circumcision scar or any genital or reproductive tract complications are likely to interfere with vaginal delivery or create problems during labor.

Situation 1: Pregnancy with Type I or II

If the circumcision is of Type I or II with a well-healed scar and no complications, no special measures or treatment will be necessary. It is sufficient to reassure the patient that she is under no special risk and to invite her to ask any questions about her circumcision or any other aspect of her health. During follow-up visits the clinician may gently inquire if she needs to speak to someone about any aspect of her health relating to circumcision. You may also find an occasion to ask about her satisfaction with her sexual relationship and inform her that specialized counseling could be made available to her. If patient literature is available you may give her a brochure in a language she can read. You do not need to do anything else unless she asks for further information or services.

Situation 2: Pregnancy with Type III (Infibulation)

If the circumcision is of Type III (infibulation), defibulation will be necessary to remove the obstruction in front of the vaginal opening. Protocols for the timing of defibulation and the counseling and consent procedures that accompany it will vary among practitioners; it is of utmost importance that your institution or practice carefully considers your particular choices. Clinically, it is most prudent not to subject the woman to extra pain or an increased possibility of infection and bleeding during labor. For this reason, the optimum time for a defibulation may be the second trimester under local anesthesia. Despite the absence of risk to the pregnancy, you may want to obtain a waiver of responsibility for any subsequent disruption to the pregnancy. If a woman is in labor and she is still infibulated, you should defibulate during the second stage of labor after the head crowns.

Counseling Against Re-infibulation

Re-infibulation (or re-stitching the cut skin hood back together), with the consent of the adult woman, is not illegal in the U.S. However it is highly undesirable from a medical point of view since it could cause obstruction to urinary flow and vaginal secretions. Every effort should be made to counsel the woman, her partner and her family against it. In countries where defibulation has been made illegal such as the U.K. there is concern that clinicians may only clarify the position of the law and do not make adequate provisions to counsel the woman regarding her feelings. Acceptance of her genitals in a state different from what she is familiar with is a status the woman has to be helped to reach with a combination of sensitive counseling and appropriate clinical care.

Counseling on re-infibulation must start at the time of discussing defibulation. The first course of action is to explain to the woman why it is better for her not to be stitched closed again. In many situations a condensed form of counseling regarding the medical risks of re-infibulation may be sufficient for her to choose not to undergo the procedure. For some women, more time is needed to think through these ideas, and you should allow for trust to develop over time. It is advisable that services and institutions providing care for infibulated women develop a counseling protocol and preferably assign a nurse or social worker who becomes knowledgeable in how to approach different communities and situations.

Experience in the Department of Obstetrics and Gynecology of the University of Aarhus in Denmark with Somali refugees shows that 90% of women decide not to undergo re-infibulation after minimal counseling with medical information. Similar results were obtained in services to Somali women in Sweden. Husbands are often (but not always) allies in convincing the woman against the procedure. For this group, mothers-in-law and other elderly women are the ones most resistant to change and should be limited in the negotiation as much as possible.

It is important to remember that the woman has known her genitals most of her life in the closed or covered form and may find it hard, both psychologically and physically, to accept a new shape and feeling to her genitals. Some women express repulsion with the softer moist parts of the exposed mucous membranes, while others experience tenderness and pain when the long-covered sensitive parts are exposed. Many express a feeling of being "naked" which was difficult to adjust to. All these issues must be taken into consideration while counseling against re-infibulation.

The patient's feelings, fears and apprehensions must be respected and addressed with compassion. Her concerns regarding physical problems or sexual ramifications must be dealt with. Some women's concern for their husband's attitude towards them, including fear of divorce, must be brought to the surface and dealt with, including fears about their husband's opinion which may be well-founded or imagined. A separate counseling session with the husband alone to ascertain his opinion and to supply him with the medical facts is advisable if the situation requires it. A third session with the couple together may follow to facilitate their communication and reach a mutual understanding and decision.

If the defibulation was done during labor, and the patient is uncertain about re-infibulation and your beliefs are against performing the procedure, it could be explained that it may be possible to have it done later if she chooses. The question remains whether the same physician or service will be willing to provide her with that option if she decides to re-infibulate and who will pay any extra costs. It is important not to give the woman insufficient or misleading information.

If she is not satisfied with that proposal and insists on immediate re-infibulation after delivery, each individual physician will have to decide what she or he is personally and professionally comfortable doing. In countries where re-infibulation is not illegal, medical advice against re-infibulation is binding neither to the health care provider nor to the patient. For the health care provider, this is probably one of the most difficult decisions to make when managing a circumcised woman. In the rare cases where the patient insists on re-infibulation despite repeated counseling the physician has three possible courses of action: 1) s/he may abstain from performing the procedure on the basis of professional and personal ethics, 2) s/he may choose to undertake a procedure that carries minimal risk (such as partial re-stitching without causing obstruction) if s/he judges it to be in the best interest of the patient, or 3) if the provider is comfortable, the woman can be referred to another provider willing to perform a minimum risk procedure.

OBSTETRICAL CARE OF CIRCUMCISED WOMEN

CHAPTER 4

41

The timing of the defibulation should be decided in consultation with the woman and her companion, if appropriate, once you have thoroughly explained her clinical risks and options. This is also the ideal time to start counseling against re-infibulation. If she (or her companion) are showing hesitation or if there is no adequate time for appropriate counseling on these points, refer her for specialized counseling. Once the patient is successfully defibulated the progress of her pregnancy and delivery should not be different from a patient who has not been circumcised.

Situation 3: Pregnancy with Local Complications

There are local complications that may affect the outcome of delivery or create complications. Large keloids or a dermoid cyst that may cause obstruction of the vaginal outlet may require surgical removal. Infected mucosal ulcers, cysts or chronic urinary tract infection may need to be drained and cleared with antibiotic treatment. Whatever the local problem, the earlier it is handled the better as long as the treatment does not interfere with the safety of the pregnancy or the health of the fetus. Adequate explanation of the situation and of any procedure to be performed is necessary to address the patient's concerns about the status of her genitals and future effects on her fertility, sexuality and marriage.

Presentation and Care of FC/FGM During Labor

Although many of the physical and counseling situations are ideally handled during pre-natal care, the delivery table may be the place where a nurse or physician first examines a circumcised woman. If you have never seen a circumcised woman or are unsure of what to do consult with a colleague who may have some experience. Prepare yourself by reading chapter 1 of this manual to familiarize yourself with the type of FC/FGM you are facing. Once the type is established read the sections of this chapter explaining the course of action to be taken for pregnancy and delivery with each type.

Assuring the woman that the clinician is knowledgeable about circumcision and is confident in managing her situation is the most important message you can convey to her. If she is infibulated, you will need to find the appropriate time and privacy to explain that defibulation is necessary for vaginal delivery, and begin counseling against re-infibulation as described above.

Under no circumstance should a woman be subjected to caesarean section solely to avoid defibulation, regardless of whether she requests it or the provider suggests it.

Post-Partum Follow-up and Counseling

Women with Type I or II circumcision will have similar postpartum needs as other women. Follow the patient's lead regarding offering her the option of sexual or psychological counseling specific to her circumcision, and do not impose it on her or ignore it regardless of her needs. The postpartum needs of women with infibulation (Type III) are similar to other women, except for special care needed for the defibulation wound.

Technique of Defibulation

Given the simplicity of the procedure defibulation can be performed under local or regional anaesthesia. However some patients may experience flash backs to the original cutting which could be psychologically painful and traumatic. A full assessment should be made in each case and the woman consulted regarding her options and preferences.

For the local anaesthesia procedure, one or two fingers (index or index and middle) are gently inserted under the hood of skin anteriorly. Local anaesthetic (such as Lidocaine) is injected along a line of skin stretched between the fingers. Extra injections of Lidocaine may be applied on the right and left of the central line. The blunt end of bandage scissors are then inserted in front of the fingers and the skin is cut anteriorly for 2–3 inches. Care

must be taken not to injure intact parts of the clitoris that may be buried under the anterior part of the hood. The cut edges are then inspected for bleeding and any excess bleeding is stopped with hemostatic (artery) forceps. The edges of the skin hood are then stitched apart with a running absorbable, non-reactive suture.

If defibulation is being performed during the course of delivery and since the course of labor cannot be ascertained until the end of the second stage it is not wise to perform defibulation until the head (or breech) is pushing against the hood of skin. In some cases where the scar has caused inelasticity of the skin around the vagina a postero-lateral episiotomy may be needed in addition to the defibulation. After the head or (breech) is delivered together with the

rest of the body, the placenta delivered, and the umbilical cord clamped, it is time to attend to the defibulation scar with hemostasis and running absorbable sutures.

Post-Defibulation Care

Local care for the vulval area is necessary for 2–4 weeks. Many women report increased sensitivity in the vulval area which was covered by the hood of skin. Sitz baths (warm water and salt) or oatmeal baths three times a day followed by gentle drying of the area and application of a soothing local cream can be prescribed for 1–2 weeks. Preparing a woman for the possibility of this temporary sensitivity and reassuring her that it will disappear should shorten the recovery time. abstinence from sexual intercourse for 4–6 weeks is also advisable.

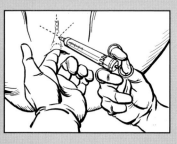
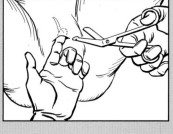
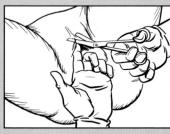
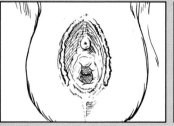
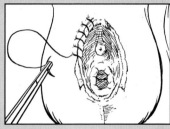
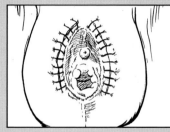

Jim Thorpe for RainbO

If the woman has not made a final decision regarding re-infibulation, a few sessions of counseling before she makes a choice should be offered.

If re-infibulation is performed, it must be insured that appropriate healing of the scar occurs and no obstruction to the flow of urine and vaginal blood results. The woman should be offered, but not forced or intimidated, to take up counseling if she so wishes. Whatever a woman's decision, she should not be made to feel bad or disapproved of.

If the newborn is a girl the family can be provided with a brochure on the harmful effects of female circumcision and its legal status in the country. A counseling session with a nurse or social worker may be arranged to provide similar information and answer the parents' questions.

Chapter 5   HEALTH CARE NEEDS OF CIRCUMCISED CHILDREN AND ADOLESCENTS

Pediatric Presentation

Most likely, the circumcision of a child is discovered accidentally during a routine check-up or treatment of a common childhood illness. The circumcised genitals of a child may, understandably, evoke much stronger feelings from the medical staff than the same in an adult. Remember this ritual was not done as a violence or as a deliberate act to hurt the child. It is a culturally normalized procedure that is deeply believed to be in the interest of the child. The parents who Westerners may perceive as cruel or abusive might have gone to great trouble and financial sacrifice to provide what they believe is their daughter's right to this ritual. They are more likely to be loving rather than abusive parents. It is important that the family is treated with respect and their right to privacy ensured. Harsh and confrontational exchanges would not be beneficial for the child nor for the reputation of the health facility.

The chances are that the girl was circumcised before she emigrated from her homeland. However, given the increasing flow of immigrants and refugees from countries where FC/FGM is prevalent, some girls may have been circumcised just before arrival. This is becoming more true as news of the illegality of the practice in the host country reaches indigenous countries. In such cases health care providers may come across children with recent circumcisions or their complications and it is not always easy to determine whether the circumcision took place in sending or receiving country. If it occurred in the host country, it is illegal in the U.S. under the federal criminal statute and may be illegal and reportable under state child abuse/protection statutes. This is also the case in all Western countries regardless of whether there is a specific FC/FGM law or it can be persecuted under general laws prohibiting bodily injury. If it was performed just prior to arrival, it is outside the jurisdiction of the criminal law in the U.S. or any other host country and is probably not reportable under child abuse/protection laws since no further harm to the child is likely. However, if a health care provider can infer from an older child's circumcision that a younger child is at risk, reporting may be warranted. (See Chapter 8 for more detailed information.)

Families who are already in the U.S. may decide to take the child to another country to be circumcised. This act is not covered by federal and state statutes criminalizing the practice in the U.S., but whether Federal authorities will deem such acts to violate child abuse and protection statutes is still unclear. If a health care provider learns of a parent's intent to circumcise the child, he or she should consider the applicability of a health provider's reporting obligations under state child abuse and protection laws. In some countries, such as Sweden, a bill is being considered that will allow persecution of individuals performing or contributing to FC/FGM on a child residing in that country even if the procedure was performed in another country, and regardless of whether it is illegal in the country where it is performed or not.

Management

Complications in a recently performed circumcision will most likely be due to infection, continued bleeding, or urine retention from severe pain or inflammation.

- Infection should be treated with systemic antibiotics and local wound care.

- Secondary bleeding from an infected hematoma of the clitoral artery can be stopped with a figure 8 stitch around the artery under general anaesthesia.

- Urinary retention can usually be overcome with pain relief and sitting the patient in warm water. On rare occasions catheterization may be necessary for a few days until the infection is controlled.

Long-term complications are likely to be the same as those encountered in adults (e.g. urethral and vaginal obstruction, dermoid cysts, ulcers, stones, etc.) and can be treated along similar lines with special attention to parental consent as a prerequisite for defibulation.

Another consideration is to arrange for psychological counseling for the child to help her overcome the effects of the trauma.

Reporting of FC/FGM in Children

While the clinician must register everything she or he finds in the patient's notes, the question of whether to report the family to social services or the legal authorities is another matter. The issue of the health care provider's duty to report a child who has undergone the procedure or who is at risk for it is governed by state laws on child abuse and protection. (See Chapter 8 for situation-specific legal considerations.) In all cases it would be appropriate to refer the case to the social worker or the community outreach worker for further counseling of the family against circumcision of this girl or her sisters. It is strongly advised that health facilities at the national regional or local level devise protocols on how to handle child reporting and protection issues.

How to Respond to a Request for Circumcision

Some health care providers will be faced with a request from a newly delivered mother or a family to circumcise their daughter. This has been a dilemma reported by nurses in post-natal wards in the U.S. when they refuse to circumcise the baby girl but agree to or even offer a circumcision for a baby boy. This creates confusion in the mind of the mother regarding the health and legal systems in America. The most important thing to do is to not react harshly or in a dismissive manner, but to use this opportunity to educate the family and help protect the child.

The physician's first response should be something like this:

'I understand that female circumcision is commonly performed in your culture and has been an old tradition. Recently there have been many studies and information from African

countries to show that this practice is harmful to girls and women. Because of that the United States (or other Western country) government together with other governments and the United Nations decided that female circumcision must be made illegal. As a health care provider in the United States I will be breaking the law if I perform this procedure and can be put in jail. You should also know that if you get it done by someone else both you and the circumciser will be subject to imprisonment and possibly deportation. Circumcision for boys is not thought to be harmful as is circumcision for girls and therefore is not illegal in America.'

The following general rules can help guide the health care provider's conversation with the parents.

- It is important to speak in a way that shows that you understand where the family comes from and that you will not condemn or judge them for asking you.

- Take this opportunity to inform them of some of the harmful effects of FC/FGM on the girl's physical and mental health, her adjustment to a new society and later her sexuality, including within marriage. Do not recite the physical complications common in Africa since they are unlikely to happen in an American (or Western) hospital or clinic and cannot be used as the justification for refusing their request.

- If the parents mention sending the child to their country of origin to be circumcised, remind them that they are putting their daughter through tremendous and unnecessary physical risk. Bring to their attention that they should think of what their daughter will feel growing up in the new country feeling so different and possibly ashamed when her friends at school learn about her circumcision. Also bring it to their attention that they may still be persecuted under child protection laws or may be made to pay civil damages to the girl or organizations working against FC/FGM in the future under a civil suit.

- Remind them that adherence to culture or preservation of virginity cannot be forced by circumcision and they are better off spending more time understanding their daughter's experience growing up in the West and talking to her about the parts of their culture she should be proud of.

- If you have no time for counseling make sure you refer the parents to a counselor (a nurse or social worker) who is familiar with the subject. On one hand, it may not be necessary to create alarm if the family can be convinced through counseling in your clinic. On the other hand, if there is reason to be concerned that the child may be at risk, it is advisable, and may be your legal duty, to alert social services so that the agency can keep in close touch with the family and take action to protect the child if necessary.

- Please note (and remind them) that FC/FGM is not a requirement of any religion, though it may be interpreted to be so by different individuals or local religious leaders.

- Provide them with brochures on the health, religious and legal aspects of FC/FGM if you have them and any other information on local community organizations working against the practice.

Special Concerns of Adolescents

Adolescent girls who have been circumcised and are living in host countries may or may not be experiencing problems particularly related to FC/FGM. Although there are no studies on the experience of circumcised adolescents growing up in the West, there is enough anecdotal evidence that their concerns about circumcision are very much intertwined with other concerns common to all adolescents regarding sexuality, body image, attractiveness, identity, belonging, and conforming with peers. Girls may have gone through the ritual at a young age in the home country; they may have clear memories of it, or may have vague or no memory of it at all, particularly if it was never discussed in the family. Girls who were not aware that they had been circumcised may find out while examining themselves, or they may suspect that they had been circumcised because of information they heard in the media or from peers. The most important thing to remember is that these young women are not dissimilar to all other teens and they require at least the same services.

A health care practitioner may become aware that a girl has undergone FC/FGM in the context of a totally unrelated matter. For example, in the course of contraceptive counseling with the school nurse or counselor, the young woman may mention that she is circumcised. In such an encounter, it is advisable to gently probe the subject and let the young woman know that she should feel comfortable talking about it if she desired. It is important to note, however, that one must not conclude from the single fact that a girl has undergone FC/FGM that she is necessarily experiencing related emotional and psychological problems. For many women, female circumcision is a part of a culture they subscribe to and accept and may not be troubled by it. Health care professionals must be extremely careful not to make these young women feel that they are viewed and treated as "abnormal." Most adolescents are more comfortable "fitting in" with the rest of their peers than "standing out." If they do not reveal any FC/FGM related problems, treating them as "different" or "abnormal" will most likely inhibit them from expressing their concerns, and may add to their load of worries and anxieties shared by most adolescents.

Alternatively, an adolescent girl may indeed be experiencing difficulties related to FC/FGM. If an adolescent girl was sexually active or considering becoming so, she may be very confused about how she may be different from her non-circumcised friends. She may present her problem to the school nurse or counselor, or seek advice from a physician. While there can be some physical problems that need attending to, the majority of adolescents will need sensitive and appropriate counseling. Peer support groups for adolescent girls who have undergone FC/FGM may be ideal mechanisms in that they provide the atmosphere of shared experience necessary for reaching out, addressing and resolving adolescent issues. (For more discussion on sexuality issues specifically relevant to circumcised women, see section 3.)

The greatest dilemma for these young women is that they fall between the values and demands of two different cultures. Part of them relates to their parents who accepted FC/FGM at least at some point in their lives but who are also likely to have traditional values which discourages sex outside of marriage. Another part may be attracted to the culture that surrounds them, which not only rejects FC/FGM but is also saturated with messages that push young people to be sexually active regardless of marriage. The resulting communication gap is often devastating to the family, particularly to the daughters. Immigrant and refugee service providers and youth counselors need to pay much more attention to this problem and find means of facilitating dialogue between adolescents and their parents to reduce family tensions. Counselors who are culturally competent to deal with adolescents from minority backgrounds must be identified, trained and encouraged to develop and share their skills with other professionals.

Young women who have been infibulated may want to seek defibulation. The health care provider must pay extra attention to issues of confidentiality in these cases to protect the adolescents privacy and safety. It is important to be aware of the possible legal and professional repercussions of providing such services to a minor without parental consent. The balance between protecting the privacy of the girl and abiding by applicable legal requirements may be a very delicate one and health facilities may want to give extra thought as to how they handle such situations.

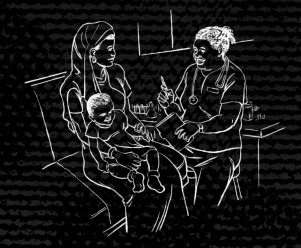

Chapter 6

INTERACTING WITH CIRCUMCISED WOMEN: SUCCESSFUL COMMUNICATION TOOLS

Cultural competence in health care has been defined as:

"The ability of individuals and systems to respond respectfully and effectively to people of all cultures, in a manner that affirms the worth and preserves the dignity of individuals, families and communities."

From "Six Steps Towards Cultural Competence: How to meet the health care needs of immigrants and refugees" *Refugee Health Program*; Minneapolis, Minnesota 1996.

A   Basics for Successful Communication

Successful medical treatment of women with FC/FGM is predicated on successful communication. Perhaps as with no other clinical situation is there a greater need for the health care provider to be culturally aware and attuned to the social and psychological circumstances of the patient. This chapter is designed to help the clinician acquire the communication skills necessary to achieve a successful medical outcome in this special patient population. Ultimately, providers must make their own assessments of the community they are serving and develop their own rapport with patients.

The health care provider has the opportunity to educate patients by providing accurate information, and positive reproductive health care experiences. Physicians, nurses and midwives are in a unique position to influence circumcised women's perceptions of themselves, their bodies and their decision to seek future health care. Some women may seek no more than standard OB/GYN services, while others may have special needs related to their circumcision, such as family planning information and appropriate birth control methods.

Effective communication is contingent on a two-way dialogue between provider and patient. The provider's own beliefs, values, and culture will influence the patient-provider interaction, and will affect interpretation of a woman's verbal and non-verbal signals. It is imperative that the provider remains nonjudgmental regardless of his or her personal beliefs and tries to find means to dialogue that facilitate the exchange of information on an equal basis.

The following are general guidelines to help you establish successful communication with circumcised women and their families:

Establish the basic facts

Given the private and sensitive nature of the practice, most women do not want information about their circumcision to be public knowledge. It is therefore inappropriate to have a question on circumcision included in the history-taking form if it will be filled by a receptionist or other non-medical staff.

Given the diversity of factors that determine the chances a woman may be circumcised, a nurse or physician trained around this issue should be able to judge if and when to ask a woman about circumcision. The question should be part of the clinician's routine history-taking, posed in the same casual tone, and not asked in isolation. If a gynecological examination is to be conducted during the visit the question may be posed just prior to asking her to lie on the examination table. For example, the clinician may say, "Before I examine you, is there anything special I need to be aware of like any previous surgery in the area or circumcision?"

Usually it is not useful to ask the patient about the type of circumcision she has unless there is a particular reason why she may know. In general, women are not familiar with the official classifications and may never have had the opportunity to view their genitals or hear a description of uncircumcised genitalia. To document the extent of her circumcision, it is best to wait for a physical examination when you can view and classify the circumcision according to standard WHO classification (see chapter 1) and enter it appropriately in the notes.

Use the right terminology

This clinical manual is not the appropriate place to explore the political debates that surround different terms such as female circumcision, genital cutting and genital mutilation. Your purposes as a clinician are better served by using language that will be most comfortable to your patients. Start by remembering not to use "genital mutilation" with patients. The majority of women prefer the term "circumcision" when speaking in English. They may be offended when they are referred to as "mutilated" or when their parents or culture are referred to as "mutilators."

In many cases women may not be familiar with the terminology in English and the best way to refer to the procedure is to use the word in her own language. Please refer to the appendices for a list of commonly used terms from various ethnic groups and languages. Even when you have used "circumcision" as a way of introducing the subject take the opportunity to ask the woman what term she prefers to use and enter it in the patient's records for future reference. (See also Appendix I.)

Secure privacy and confidentiality for the client

Once it is established that the woman is circumcised, the information, and the subsequent clinical examination should be handled with professionalism and discretion. Avoid whispering and gazing amongst the staff, expressing pity or exhibiting patronizing attitudes. The nurse or physician should convey to the patient that s/he is comfortable dealing with her condition. It is neither appropriate nor productive to display any feelings of horror or disapproval to the woman. Staff who have been educated and trained beforehand are best prepared to handle the patient, and will be less likely to react inappropriately. The patient should be made to feel confident that she is in safe hands, will not be judged and will not be made an object of curiosity or put on display. The most traumatizing experience women have reported is when a woman's circumcision was first discovered during a pelvic examination by a health care provider unfamiliar with the practice who then called in the rest of the staff to look at her "mutilated" genitals.

"The feeling of vulnerability and shame I felt lying on my back naked with my legs open and being reduced to a curious spectacle on public display is something I will never forget. It is worse than what I remember of the circumcision."

Regardless of any educational justification, a woman must not be viewed or examined by any staff other than the attending physician and nurse unless she consents to be part of a teaching session. The clinician should emphasize that care is not conditional on the woman's consent to an educational session. Also, unless she requires it or translation necessitates it, no other person should be present at the time of examination or during further questioning about her circumcision. It is of utmost importance that the patient's right to privacy and confidentiality is rigorously protected. The fact that she may be unfamiliar with Western health systems, speak a different language and have an unusual condition is no excuse to violate her rights.

Do not stereotype your patient

In the United States, it is still common for individuals to be referred to as Africans or from the Middle East, obscuring a wide variety of social, cultural, religious and individual differences. For example, individuals from the same region, or even country, may be Christian, Muslim or belong to a local religion. Within each religion and culture there are social variations which affect an individual's behavior and choices. For example the way a woman chooses to dress should not be used as a license for you to define who she is. The common stereotype of a Muslim woman—veiled, passive and submissive—will not fit all Muslim women you will meet; and a woman dressed in traditional dress such as the boubou common to West Africans may be a housewife, a University lecturer or a street vendor.

When addressing women or referring to them, it is a matter of respect to address them by name or refer to them, for example, according to the color of their clothing such as "the lady wearing the pink silk dress" rather than using such potentially discriminatory and objectifying terms as "that black woman" or "that African woman."

Set the right tone of interaction

When a patient walks into a health care facility, she will immediately get a sense whether she is welcome. Pictures or posters in the waiting areas that reflect the patients ethnicity or their culture will help set them at ease. If you routinely serve a particular community, you may want to learn a few greeting words from the language of the patients. It is a simple gesture that acknowledges their culture and shows that you are willing to make an effort.

A warm greeting is an expectation in most African and Middle eastern cultures and will help determine the success of any subsequent conversation. In America "Hello" is considered to be sufficient. For many Africans the greeting may involve not only the initial salutation but also a number of cordial inquiries about family. Such a greeting on the part of the physician or nurse may encourage patients to talk about what is happening in their communities. Good eye contact and a smile will reassure the patient that you treat her as an individual.

Support the woman's decision-making process

While in the U.S. and other Western cultures, women are expected to advocate for and make decisions regarding their own health, in many African cultures a woman's decision-making process is expected to involve the family. You will need to assess when a woman wants to make individual decisions or involve others. To support a woman's right to make her own decision you must provide the space for her to express her needs. If she chooses to involve her husband or family members you should also be supportive of that process.

Understand her health care behavior and practices

In many African societies physicians and nurses are held in very high esteem and thought to be very knowledgeable. They may be expected to diagnose the ailment and prescribe treatment without lengthy questioning. The patient may be reluctant to answer extensive history taking so it is important to explain to her the significance of such information. Some women may never have had a pelvic examination and may be reluctant to expose their genitals so you must explain in advance what you will be doing. Some patients may come seeking a tangible treatment such as a pill or an injection and may need longer explanation why such treatment is not necessary.

Traditional medicine plays an important role in the health seeking behavior of many African women. To most modern health care providers the use of traditional medicine is still considered a sign of ignorance. While it is true that many traditional healing methods may be harmful, others may be beneficial or inconsequential. Some African immigrants still defer to traditional medicine in the form of herbal teas and washes, scarification, cauterization, and bloodletting as home remedies or as prescribed by traditional healers. Some women may use herbs to prepare the birth canal. In addition, the belief in the evil eye is widespread among African immigrants. To protect oneself, a person may wear anklets, belts made of beads, or shells to ward off dangerous spirits. Some individuals choose a fluctuating balance between the use of traditional and modern healing systems. It is important to respect the patient's beliefs and to work with her to discourage her use of potentially harmful home remedies, particularly those which may cause drug interaction, while endorsing those which may give her physical or psychological comfort.

Give appropriate and well-timed information

When giving information, the provider should recognize that whatever is said and how it is said will influence the outcome of the treatment. To ensure the communication of adequate information the physician or nurse should:

- Make sure to speak slowly and clearly and use simple but accurate terms.

- Use pictures and diagrams as much as possible for women with low literacy.

- Do not overwhelm the patient with too much new information during the first visit; select the most important information and postpone the rest for follow-up visits.

- In urban settings or situations where the patient may not return for subsequent care, give out adequate written information.

- Ask whether she understood the most vital information necessary for her to make a decision or to follow a course of treatment and ask the patient to repeat the most important points. Give her adequate time, and encourage her to ask questions.

When taking history or asking other questions you may want to observe the following:

- Give the woman ample time to respond to questions.

- Do not interrupt her or presuppose her answers.

- Do not force her to repeat things in medical terms, or in popular American English.

- Repeat back to the patient your understanding of what she has said.

B   Barriers to Successful Communication

Language

Immigrant and refugee women identify language as one of the major barriers to seeking health care. Providing adequate interpretation is one of the requirements of the Minority Health Act of the United States. Larger hospitals and groups of clinics often consolidate their resources and create interpreter banks. Whenever possible a well trained medical interpreter should be made available to the patient. The use of family interpreters should be avoided when there are other options, even if one is voluntarily provided.

When dealing with sensitive issues of reproductive health and sexuality (including FC/FGM) the personal characteristics of the professional interpreter become exceedingly important. Professional interpreters are usually trained on issues of patient confidentiality. However, a woman's perception of the interpreter and their role may impact the exchange. A woman may not feel comfortable discussing issues related to her genitals with a professional male interpreter from her own ethnic background or from her community, or she may not want to reveal sexual or marital problems to a stranger who is not a physician. In general, with regard to reproductive health, women tend to express a preference for female interpreters even when they are indifferent to the gender of the health care provider.

While professional interpreters may be available for some languages and in areas serving larger populations, it may sometimes be difficult to provide interpretation services if the patient's language is less common, or the population served is very small. To combat this problem, some providers use call-in interpretation services such as national dial-in language lines, but the services cannot provide every language, or the costs may be prohibitive to some institutions. Though these may be useful, they are not an adequate substitute for face-to-face interpretation. When neither of the above is available, it is often unavoidable that the patient provides her own interpreter. **Always choose an adult family member as an interpreter and avoid using children.** Using children as interpreters imposes the unfair burden of taking responsibility for an adult, and inappropriately exposes the youngsters to intimate information about their elders.

When the interpreter is a family member, three main problems can arise: **1)** when a child, spouse, or other family member interprets, the imbalance of power between family members may interfere with adequate care and decision making, and may keep women from being frank with the provider; **2)** s/he is not trained in objective translation; **3)** s/he usually does not know scientific terms and is unaware of confidentiality issues.

If appropriate interpreters are not readily available, clinicians should do their best with what is available. Most important is to be aware of the possible dynamics involved in the three-way exchange and try to overcome them. **The golden rule is to "always look at and talk to the woman directly and not to her interpreter."** Meanwhile take other measures to improve the situation in future visits. For example, if the interpreter is a relative, try to find an independent interpreter for the following visit. If the interpreter is a child avoid discussing very sensitive issues at the first encounter and inquire if she can bring an adult (preferably female) interpreter for the next visit. A long-term solution may be possible by identifying women from within the community who can be trained to become patient advocates and interpreters. (This aspect of care is discussed in Chapter 7.)

Patient and/or provider modesty

Many women who come from African countries where FC/FGM is prevalent may have had a social upbringing which emphasized social and physical modesty. Some women consider it vulgar to discuss their genitals, and would not be comfortable talking about their sexuality, or sexual behavior. The clinician should welcome the patient's guidance in discussing such matters by telling her that though women are biologically the same everywhere their cultural practices differ. Ask such questions as "How do women feel about… in your culture?" which may open up the conversation in a less personalized way.

Clinicians should assess their own beliefs and values regarding such private issues, and recognize that his/her own sense of modesty may contribute to any unease sensed when approaching subjects of reproductive health. With appropriate training in sexual counseling, and gentle probing into the patient's own comfort level during the clinical encounter, the clinician should be able to build trust over time to overcome this universal obstacle.

Perceptional differences

One of the least recognized difficulties of communication between patient and provider is the difference in knowledge and perceptions regarding bodily functions and therefore what constitutes appropriate health care. The patient comes from a cultural context that assigns bodily functions based on knowledge that is not derived from biomedical science. Health care providers are trained in Western style biomedicine sometimes mixed with their own cultural perceptions.

One incident that illustrates this is a dialogue that occurred between OB/GYN staff (nurse-midwives and physicians) in a European setting and a group of refugee women they served. The refugee women were infibulated, and complained that they were not given adequate support during their labor and were instructed to keep pushing. The providers explained that they followed their usual procedure and gave uterine contractors (oxytocin) whenever necessary and routinely performed defibulation to facilitate the second stage of labor. On further probing it was clarified that the practice in the women's community involves another woman sitting behind her encircling her with her arms for support as she is pushing. Since they were not receiving such physical support, the women thought their bodies were "tearing inside" because they were infibulated. They were unaware that since they are defibulated there is no further risk of tearing and that their "inside" is not affected by the infibulation. This example demonstrates two very different perceptions and approaches to solutions. The medical doctors were clear about the physiological and anatomical facts and used biomedical solutions of defibulation and uterine contractors to facilitate labor. The women were protesting the lack of combined physical and emotional support necessary to address their perception of their abnormal bodies with an embrace that also protected them from the memories of their initial trauma.

How does one resolve this difference between medical and cultural perceptions? First take the time to explain what exactly was cut when she was circumcised and what you are doing to minimize the effect on her labor. When necessary, show her simple diagrams of normal and infibulated anatomy, the physiology of labor and how—for the purposes of delivery their circumcision could be reversed with defibulation. Second, look into the possibility of allowing a female friend or relative to attend labor to give the customary support. With careful listening, the problems can be identified and solutions found.

Physician-Patient-Family power dynamics

When interacting with a patient from another culture there are at least two belief systems which must be dealt with: the clinician's and the patient's. If the woman is accompanied by her husband, mother-in-law or male relative her own opinions and needs may become secondary to theirs. Negotiating the gender and power dynamics between the woman and her family, and between the clinician and the woman within a comfort zone of both sets of beliefs is a formidable task. Women's needs and choices will fall at opposite ends of the spectrum and anywhere in between. Some will not deal with a health care provider without the presence of a male relative and may defer decisions to him. In this case, the clinician must respect her comfort level and include others in her decision-making while constantly referring to her for her opinion. Another woman may welcome the chance to ask questions and make independent choices for herself. This woman may appreciate a private session without family members. In recognizing, respecting and working within these dynamics, the clinician should be able to tailor care so as to not create conflict between a woman and her family.

The provider's sex

One of the most commonly perceived barriers to communication is that women from non-Western countries prefer a female health care provider, particularly for reproductive health care. This is not universally true. Many women who come from societies where social modesty is important have expressed no preference for the sex of the health care provider, and believe in the neutrality of the physician. Some may even express more confidence in the wisdom and knowledge of male physicians. This may be explained by the fact that in their own countries most physicians are men. On the other hand those who have experienced female physicians often prefer them for their reproductive health care. Female nurses, midwives and interpreters are always preferred and are often seen as allies or confidantes. Most circumcised women prefer a health care provider from their own or neighboring culture, particularly if the individual can speak their language. In practice, most circumcised women are attracted to particular clinics or individual health care providers on the recommendation of other women because of the providers' sensitivity and compassion regardless of race, sex or nationality.

Should there be further discussions of circumcision or its effects?

Other questions health care providers ask are:

Q1   *Is it appropriate to talk further with a woman about her circumcision?*

Q2   *When should I talk about it?*

Q3   *What should I say?*

The answers are:

A1   *Only if it is necessary.*

A2   *When you have informed yourself and she is ready.*

A3   *Be guided by what is relevant to the patient's clinical situation and to the stage of inquiry she is in.*

If her clinical condition is related to her circumcision, you obviously need to explain the situation. For example, if she has a complication related to her circumcision such as a cyst or an infection, you should explain what caused it and what procedure may be necessary to treat it. Also, if she is infibulated and pregnant, defibulation will have to be discussed at some point. Defibulation and re-infibulation are discussed in detail in Chapter 4. If her clinical condition is not affected by her circumcision, there is no need to discuss the matter any further, particularly during the first visit, unless she clearly expresses a desire to do so.

If the patient indicates no problem and the clinician still feels the need to talk further about her circumcision, it may be useful for the clinician to examine his or her own motives. It is inappropriate to pursue questioning to satisfy personal curiosity or express a personal point of view. The clinician is better advised to read further on the subject, discuss it with knowledgeable colleagues or contact local community organizations.

Some health care providers report that at some point during the clinical care it becomes obvious that some women would benefit from looking at a drawing of the shape of their genitals or actually viewing their own vulval area with a mirror. This should not be offered in a first or early visit but should be kept in mind as a possibility. Sometimes looking at her own genitals in a mirror can demystify the problem and give the woman a sense of re-owning her body. This approach is not suitable for all women and could be traumatizing if not used judiciously.

The most important rule is to follow the patient's leads and closely monitor her comfort zone. The clinician should convey the message that he/she is available to talk but will not pursue the subject if the patient is not ready. Like many other situations it is fine judgement and delicate balance which make for a good clinician. As the relationship between provider and patient develops the opportunity will arise to talk about her knowledge and views of circumcision, inform her about its damaging effects and its legal status in the country. One way to prepare for the discussions is to provide her with written information in the form of patient literature. You may also refer her to a community support group or a counselor. (See chapter 7.)

Counseling

In many African societies the concept of health encompasses both the physical and psychological, each reinforcing the other. When a patient seeks the help of a healer, she is most likely prompted by physical symptoms. However, in the traditional healing practices of most African cultures, a healer does not simply dispense herbs or prescribe treatment; s/he also provides counseling to the patients. In addition to discussing the presenting physical symptoms, the treatment may include discussions of the patient's life—daily activities, past and present events. Hence, when treatment is prescribed, the healer has not only dealt with the physical aspects of the problem, but has also helped alleviate the patient's fears, worries or concerns. In some cases, the healer even acts as a mediator between couples or family members, still in the context of treating the patient. The patient is therefore able to discuss her emotional or psychological problems without the social stigma often attached to mental illness.

For many Africans, specialized counseling or mental health services—as may be practiced in the West—may seem alien or strange, particularly when the mental and physical are treated separately. In many African countries psychology as a science has not gained much attention in medical facilities; the few specialists in the field only have time to deal with extremely debilitating mental illnesses.

Consequently, little has been known of the everyday psychological effects of circumcision on a girl or a woman and even less about possible approaches to provide counseling on FC/FGM. Most women may consider counseling as strange, or even a waste of their time.

Do all circumcised women need counseling?

The definitive answer is NO. Not all women who have been circumcised want or need counseling. Many circumcised women are very well adjusted and enjoy a healthy emotional and sexual life. On the other hand, many women who may benefit from counseling are not provided such an option, or may not know of the services that are available to them.

Assessing the client's need for counseling.

In the clinical situation, the health care provider is advised to assess the client's needs without imposing personal values and beliefs on the client. To do so, the clinician may:

- provide written information (a leaflet) about the availability and possible benefits of counseling, while leaving it up to the patient to request such services.

- mention existing support services—avoid labeling it "counseling service"—and based on the client's responsiveness, the clinician may either make the referral, or stop at letting her know that more information would be made available upon her request.

However, it is extremely important to remember that the provider must NOT make assumptions based on personal values and beliefs in assessing the woman's needs. The clinician should avoid suggesting that a woman "must be angry or suffering." It would be inappropriate to even suggest solutions to problems that may not exist to begin with. By so doing, the patient would most likely feel judged and mistreated, and may not return to the health facility.

When should circumcised women be referred for counseling?

There are cases whereby the clinician should strongly recommend, or refer a circumcised woman to counseling.

1 When a circumcised woman expresses enthusiasm for counseling or requests a referral.

2 When the clinician is convinced that counseling is necessary for a favorable outcome of the treatment. For example, an infibulated pregnant woman who may be anxious about defibulation may need counseling—including counseling against re-infibulation—since she may be experiencing flashbacks of her circumcision. Counseling is also necessary when the clinician suspects that total relief of the presenting symptoms will not be achieved with surgical or medical intervention alone and some therapeutic counseling may be necessary.

3 When the presenting symptoms are primarily psychological or sexual in nature.

Where can circumcised women receive counseling?

As the patient-provider relationship develops, the circumcised woman may request or be clearly in need of counseling services. There are three main barriers to providing this service for women:

1 Lack of mental health professionals who are familiar with cross-cultural issues.

2 Lack of knowledge of the practice of FC/FGM and its possible effect on women.

3 Reluctance by most circumcised women to speak to foreign counselors.

Institutions and professionals who service a large population of circumcised women may want to invest in gaining knowledge and experience in this area by hiring an individual who specializes in outreach and counseling for women who have been circumcised. Look for an opportunity to recruit a qualified woman from the community (for example someone with a nursing or social work degree) and provide her with training in counseling. She will add valuable cultural knowledge to your services.

Creating a counseling or support group for circumcised women is another possibility. The supportive presence of others with a similar experience may help reduce the woman's suspicion and anxiety towards counseling. Such a group will, in turn, increase knowledge and awareness of the psychological needs and feelings of those who have to live with circumcision. The group facilitator must bear in mind the diversity within the African immigrant community, particularly among circumcised women, in terms of culture, language, education, age and marital status and how that may affect the group dynamic. It may be advisable to start support and counseling groups with individuals with similar characteristics to encourage openness and avoid conflict.

Other institutions and professionals who may encounter circumcised women less frequently may want to be prepared by researching if other health care institutions offer counseling for circumcised women. Moreover, although community based organizations servicing populations of African immigrants may not provide counseling on FC/FGM specifically, they may be extremely helpful in locating practicing counselors or therapists from within the community who are familiar with the subject. They may also want to introduce FC/FGM to their existing support groups.

Reproductive Health Education

Many women do not have access to reproductive and sexual health information and may not have seen a diagram of the reproductive organs, or normal female genitals. Many circumcised women may not have an understanding of the type of circumcision they have. Providing such information within the limited time available at the clinical session is almost impossible.

Educational Workshops

Hospitals and clinics that service communities with large numbers of circumcised women may consider conducting group education sessions on reproductive anatomy and physiology, general reproductive health information such as contraception and prevention of sexually transmitted disease and types of circumcisions performed on women. Such sessions could be incorporated into pre-natal care services, school and women's health clinics, maternal and infant care programs and other venues where groups of women may gather. Because in some cultures women may shy away from publicly discussing reproductive health aspects, it would be advisable during outreach to refer to it in a more comprehensive title such as "Women's Health."

Development of Educational Material

The preparation of simple and clear material in print that can be available in waiting rooms and postnatal wards could also add to the information available to women. As much as possible this material should be made available in English and other languages of the populations served such as French, Arabic, Somali, Amharic and Swahili.

Because of the complex cultural variables involved in receiving and processing information, it is extremely important that providers engaging in the production of educational materials consult with professionals and institutions who may lend their expertise in assessing how this information should be presented to the target population. Anecdotal evidence has shown repeatedly that when educational materials were produced in the absence of cultural context, the women were not able to relate to or process the information. The contribution of community-based organizations, research centers, resource persons and professionals from the communities will greatly determine how well the educational materials may be received by the women.

Outreach

Since only a fraction of circumcised women actually come in contact with health services, some health programs, social services, and refugee resettlement agencies may consider incorporating FC/FGM information and educational efforts in their work. The first step to take is to sensitize the program or service staff to the needs of circumcised women and identify the barriers women may face in accessing services and information.

Hospitals and health care providers may consider engaging in partnerships with community-based organizations and other service providers for African immigrants in order to reach a wider population than the fraction that voluntarily seeks health care. Such partnerships could involve projects such as the training of health care provider staff on cultural sensitivity by the community based organizations and/or workshops for immigrant women on select aspects of health and the health care system of the host country. A hospital or other health care provider may collaborate by sponsoring an event organized by a community-based organization, such as community health fairs targeting African immigrant women.

Institutions and agencies with the resources to provide training for community health educators may also want to invest in recruiting women from the community. Experience shows that the most successful outreach staff are those who are part of the community since women respond to them faster than to outsiders. In addition, setting up such a program will provide employment opportunities for immigrant women who are usually motivated to serve their own community.

Access

Given that the majority of circumcised women are first generation refugees and immigrants, they all face numerous barriers to accessing health care. As mentioned in Chapter 6, language is one of the well-identified barriers to accessing of health care services. Hospitals and clinics serving large numbers of patients with a particular language should consider recruiting and training patient companions and translators from within the community, particularly other women. Resources should be made available to employ or remunerate these individuals rather than rely on the use of their time as volunteers.

In Europe, Canada, and Australia where health care is a universal right to all who are legally residing in the country, there are no financial barriers to accessing the health care system. However, cultural and communication barriers still operate in limiting circumcised women from accessing health care.

In the United States, access to health care is generally limited by insurance coverage or one's ability to pay, and most recently by a person's immigration status. With the cuts in social benefits to legal immigrants—many of whom have low income—it is important to consider ways to facilitate low cost and subsidized care for circumcised women. Health care providers and institutions can help in overcoming this barrier by identifying existing public services that are available, including not-for-profit, private and charity clinics that provide services on a sliding scale, and then making the information widely available.

Moreover, in the U.S., lack of transportation to health care facilities is another barrier to accessing services. Since the private car is the major mode of transport in most locations with the exception of a few major cities, immigrant and refugee women are handicapped since most do not know how to drive nor have the linguistic skills to obtain a driver's license. Facilitating transportation for women may be another consideration when attempting to improve access to health care.

A final barrier to access experienced by many immigrant and refugee women is the lack of childcare at home. Hospitals and clinics may consider incorporating childcare centers in their services as part of facilitating access to care for women.

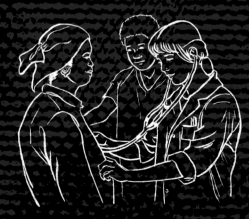

Chapter 8

THE LAW AND FEMALE CIRCUMCISION

Due to the general nature of the discussion contained in this chapter, it should not be regarded as legal advice. If you have any questions, please consult an attorney. Institutional providers may wish to consult with their legal departments.

The social, cultural and economic explanations for FC/FGM in this manual are not meant to justify or apologize for the practice. Whatever the reasons, the end result is that a child is subjected to a painful and physically unnecessary procedure which has the potential of causing lasting physical and psychological harm.

For immigrants and refugees the social and economic context that compelled parents to circumcise their daughters no longer exists and the only lasting reason for the practice is to preserve cultural identity. In a modern legal system that seeks to protect the rights of each individual, "culture" is no longer acceptable as a justification for violating the bodily integrity of a child by removing a healthy part of her body or performing any other ritual that may be detrimental to her mental or physical health. Prompted by activists from both the northern countries and Africa, the international community including the World Health Organization and the UN Commission on Human Rights, began to condemn the practice of FC/FGM as a violation of internationally recognized human rights. At the national level, laws have been passed criminalizing the practice in countries receiving African immigrants—such as Australia, Norway, Sweden, and the United Kingdom—as well as in some African countries such as Ghana (1994), Burkina Faso (1996), Cote d'Ivoire[Ivory Coast], Togo and Senegal (1998). (See Appendix IV, p. 94.) In Egypt a ministerial decree issued in 1997 prohibits the practice and makes it punishable under existing laws of grievous bodily injury.

Legal Status in the U.S.

A federal law criminalizing FGM was passed in 1996 and became effective in April 1997. (See Appendix II, p. 87.) This law provides that performing FC/FGM in the United States on a girl under age 18 is a felony punishable by fines or up to 5 years imprisonment. The statute provides that "whoever knowingly circumcises, excises, or infibulates the whole or any part of the labia majora or labia minora or clitoris of another person" under 18 is guilty under the statute. The statute exempts a surgical operation that is "necessary to the health of the person on whom it is performed, and is performed by a person licensed in the place of its performance as a medical practitioner." The law specifically exempts cultural beliefs or practices as a defense.

The law clearly penalizes those who perform the cutting, whether they are medically trained or not. Moreover, general principles of criminal law could extend liability to a parent, guardian, or other person (an "accomplice" or "accessory") who consents to, assists in arranging or is otherwise involved in the procedure.

Under well-established legal principles, American criminal laws do not extend beyond the territorial boundaries of the United States. Thus, circumcisions performed in other countries are not punishable under U.S. law. Moreover, federal law does not apply to procedures performed on women over age 18. Thus, adult women could consent to circumcision as they would other elective, non-medically indicated surgical procedures such as cosmetic surgery. This would include consent to re-infibulation (see below).

State Laws

As of December 1998, ten states enacted criminal laws on FC/FGM. These are California, Delaware, Illinois, Maryland, Minnesota, New York, North Dakota, Rhode Island, Tennessee and Wisconsin. These were enacted prior to and after the federal law's passage. Several additional states have introduced legislation on FC/FGM, though these bills have not yet passed. Other state legislatures may choose to address the issue in the future as well.

Most state laws take an approach similar to the federal law in criminalizing FC/FGM. Some state laws on FC/FGM—including Illinois, Minnesota, Rhode Island and Tennessee—prohibit performance of the procedure generally, without specifying an age limit. These laws thus leave open the possibility of criminalization of surgery performed on women above the age of consent. Other state laws such as California and Delaware explicitly criminalize the conduct of parents or guardians who "permit" or "allow" FC/FGM to be performed.

In states where laws on FC/FGM exist in addition to the federal law, both state and federal law enforcement authorities could bring criminal charges against individuals for violations. In addition, in states where no specific legislation related to FC/FGM has been passed, existing statutes related to child abuse/child protection; assault and battery; and/or the unlawful practice of medicine may also result in a health care provider or parent being found legally liable for his or her involvement in FC/FGM. It is worth noting that the American Medical Association specifically condemned the practice and supported the enactment of legislation to criminalize the practice in the United States. For the latest information on whether your state has a specific law on FC/FGM or a general law that may apply, consult with your legal advisers.

Why Pass Such Laws?

The U.S. Congress and various state legislatures have asserted that criminal laws are necessary in order to ensure that FC/FGM is not practiced among immigrant groups in the U.S. such that girls are compelled to suffer the often severe physical and psychological effects of the practice. Congress concluded that the "unique circumstances" surrounding the practice warranted federal legislation as it could be beyond the control of any single state or local jurisdiction to control.

Various states passed legislation before and after the federal law was passed, believing it prudent to have specific state legislation to address an issue with clear domestic relations ramifications, a sphere traditionally regulated by states. Moreover, states have traditionally had jurisdiction over torts and crimes perpetrated against the physical integrity of another. However, it has become less unusual for federal and state criminal statutes to "overlap" in their prohibitions. Thus, federal and state authorities could have jurisdiction over the same act involving FC/FGM.

A health care provider should also be aware of the following issues regarding applicable laws:

Legal Risks of Caring for Circumcised Girls and Women

While performing FC/FGM is illegal in the United States, caring for women who are already circumcised is not illegal. In fact, refusing to care for circumcised women could result in severely damaging their willingness to avail themselves of health care services. Health care providers presented with such women have a unique opportunity to positively impact these women's lives by being open to treating the complications these women suffer, if any. Of course, denying medical treatment and thereby providing inadequate care may carry malpractice risks that do not exist if appropriate care is provided.

Defibulation

Defibulation, or opening up the tightly sewn vulva of a woman with Type III FC/FGM, is not illegal and is medically encouraged as long as it is performed with the informed consent of the woman without any form of coercion. (See chapter 4 for details.) In cases where FC/FGM has already occurred and defibulation is not necessitated by a medical emergency, such as during childbirth, a clinician who performs defibulation on a girl under the age of consent without her parents' or guardian's permission may risk sanctions under state law applicable to a health care provider's failure to obtain required consent. Consult your local legal counsel for further details on the law in your state.

Re-infibulation

Re-infibulation, or closing the vulva of a woman with Type III FC/FGM after defibulation had been performed to facilitate delivery of a child, is not illegal under existing law in most states if the woman is over 18. However, while the criminal statutes on FC/FGM do not explicitly address re-infibulation, it is likely that law enforcement and judicial personnel would interpret them to prohibit a person from performing this procedure on a girl under age 18. While it is not clear whether re-infibulation constitutes part of pregnancy-related medical treatment, it is worth noting that in the case of pregnant women under 18, the law in most states considers them "exempted minors," that is, their pregnancy has rendered them legally competent to make decisions regarding their medical care without parental consent.

Experience shows that informative and respectful counseling against re-infibulation removes the conflict between the woman's cultural orientation towards re-infibulation and the physician/nurses' orientation against the procedure. Most women agree not to re-infibulate once the potential health risks are explained to them. Clearly, avoiding legal measures and judicial intervention is always desirable. If the woman insists on re-infibulation despite adequate counseling, it is then left to the physician to consider whether to follow her request or abstain from performing the procedure on the basis of professional and ethical consciousness. (See Chapter 4 for a detailed discussion of the issues related to re-infibulation.)

Reporting to the Authorities

In most states, the fact that FC/FGM is a criminal offense probably does not itself create an affirmative duty on the part of health care providers to report it in adults. However, most state laws do require physicians and other health care providers to report child abuse and suspicion of future imminent harm to the child. Thus, health care providers should review applicable state laws related to their duty to report suspected instances of child abuse and consider whether and how FC/FGM is encompassed in state legislation governing child abuse/protection. Given the cultural complexities involved, particularly the fact that parents intend to benefit, not harm, their daughters, and that the risk of future harm after FC/FGM is performed is usually nonexistent, reporting a procedure that has already occurred may not be warranted. However, if there are other uncircumcised daughters in the family or if the health care provider learns of an intended, but not yet executed, circumcision (to take place either in the U.S. or abroad), reporting may be warranted or required under state law to protect the child.

It is worth reemphasizing that parents are not liable under the criminal statutes on FC/FGM if the procedure occurred outside the territorial jurisdiction of the U.S. Extreme caution is necessary when dealing with recent refugees and immigrants, many of whom circumcise their daughters just before they come to the U.S. For those who are known to have resided in the U.S. for a longer period, the procedure may have been performed during a visit abroad. This action does not violate federal or state criminal statutes. However, if a health care provider learns that a parent intends to take the child out of the U.S. for the procedure, reporting may be warranted under state child abuse/protection laws.

If the clinician is presented with a fresh wound complication in a young girl, it is advisable for that individual and/or the social worker to assist the family to understand the legal situation in the U.S. and counsel them against the practice. As discussed above, whether there is a duty to report the FC/FGM will depend upon whether state law mandates reporting crimes generally and/or child abuse, assuming FC/FGM falls under that definition, even in circumstances when no future harm to the child is likely.

It is important to keep in mind that recently arrived refugees and immigrants often have few financial resources to spend on defending themselves. An unjustified reporting can be extremely detrimental to the well being of the whole family.

Counseling the Patient on the Law

It is possible that the patient may not have heard of the law against FC/FGM in the United States. It is the professional obligation of the physician to take the opportunity of the clinical encounter to inform the woman and her family about the law. This is best not done as the first part of the clinical exchange and time should be allowed for the woman to develop a degree of trust and appreciation for the care she is given before the law is mentioned. Experience shows that people respond better to concern for their well-being than to threats of punishment.

The passage of laws that criminalize a practice that is largely confined to new immigrants and refugees, coupled with the use of terminology favored by some rights advocates, such as "mutilation" and "barbarism" have already angered many individuals. Those in immigrant communities who come from countries where female circumcision is performed feel unjustly targeted in their new country. It is prudent to use great care in how you approach the subject because you may have to deal with anger not caused by your own words or actions.

The following line of questions and responses is one model of how you may handle counseling on the law:

Q1   *Ask whether the person knows that there is a federal law (and state, if applicable). If they do not know, explain what the law does and the basic reason for its passage, i.e. to protect the health and well-being of girl children, in as clear and easy terms as possible and provide them with legal literature if available. Refer them to your local legal aid society for more detailed information.*

   If they already are aware of the law, go to Q2.

Q2   *Ask what they think of the law.*

   If they approve, drop the subject.

   If they do not approve, proceed to Q3.

Q3   *Ask whether the person believes that FC/FGM should be stopped. If yes: Ask what they believe is the best way to stop it.*

   If no: Explain that their disapproval of the law does not exempt them from punishment if they take part in a decision to perform the procedure. If available, provide legal and other literature on the subject. The most effective information is that published by the patient's own cultural group. Also consider referring the family to an FC/FGM-informed social worker for further counseling if necessary. Document any responses or suggestions.

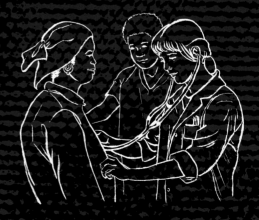

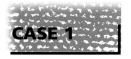

Genet is a 43 years old Ethiopian teacher who presented to
a private gynecology specialist complaining of **swelling in the vulval
area** which is causing her no pain but is increasing in size over the
years. She is not certain whether she wants it removed since she has
had it for many years. She is a little worried because it has been
growing bigger in the last few months. She volunteered the information
that she was circumcised.

Her history revealed that she was divorced, and has no current sexual
partner. She recently started dating an Ethiopian University-professor
and the relationship is getting serious.

On examination she was confirmed to have a **mild form of Type II
circumcision**; a part of the clitoris and a small part of the anterior labia
were removed. She was also found to have **a cyst attached to the left
side of the labial scar** about the size of a hazelnut. It was mildly tender
but not infected. The rest of her examination revealed no other
abnormality.

The physician explained to her that the cyst was made of a
blocked sebaceous gland and that it will not cause her any serious
complications. He offered her the option of removing it at this
time or any time in the future if it was causing her any physical or
psychological discomfort. Sensing from her body language that there
was more to her worries than the cyst he gently asked her if there were
any other issues she wanted to ask about and whether she had **other
worries related to her circumcision**.

She told him that she had left her country at the age of five when
her father became a diplomat in the 1950s. Although she had visited
several times, she had never again lived in her own country. In her
mid-twenties she married an Ethiopian student in Europe but after
the first couple of years it was clear that the marriage, and the sexual
relationship, was not successful. During this time she had become
aware of the issue of FC/FGM from the media and was not sure
she was circumcised. She was seen by several OB/GYN specialists in
Europe and the U.S. before one of them confirmed to her that indeed
she was circumcised with a Type II circumcision. When her husband
learned this fact he blamed the failure of the marriage on her
"frigidity" and they divorced. She has been living in the U.S. since
then but has not remarried or had any sexual relationship.

She confided that she is very scared of what will happen if she allowed
her relationship with the professor to become more serious and
worried that she will fail him sexually. She volunteered that she feels
confused because she finds him a very understanding and liberal man
and that he expressed his opposition to FC/FGM. After reassuring her
that she need not feel inadequate or guilty and that **she can have a
successful relationship despite her circumcision** the physician
referred her to a therapist. After a few private sessions with the
therapist Genet was able to talk to the professor about her worries.

He was very understanding and reassured her that his deceased wife was also circumcised and that they managed to have a fulfilling relationship for 20 years. The therapist arranged a few more joint sessions with the couple to help them discuss their concerns more openly and they were married a few months later. The sebaceous cyst opened spontaneously while she was having a hot bath and it never needed surgery.

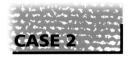

CASE 2

Salha is a 27 year old Sudanese University-student

who presented to the student's health center with symptoms of **severe dysmenorrhea and irregular menses**. She specifically requested a female clinician to examine her.

On examination she was found to have **Type III FC/FGM (infibulation)** with a tight opening over the vagina which would only allow one small finger. She was extremely tense and jumped whenever the area of her vulva were examined. The nurse practitioner (NP) explained that she needed to do a **bimanual rectal examination to feel the pelvic organs**. There was tenderness over the bladder indicating a possibility of low grade cystitis but other pelvic organs were normal.

The NP explained that she seems to have **chronic cystitis** that may be contributing to her menstrual pain and irregularity. She explained that the treatment will be a course of antibiotics after taking a urine sample for culture and that she also needed to be **defibulated to remove the obstruction in front of the urethra**.

Salha explained that she is engaged to be married to an American man who knows about her circumcision but they do not know how they will handle the wedding night. She expressed a desire to be fully defibulated together with **any other procedure that would ensure easier intercourse and more sexual satisfaction**.

The NP explained that the attending physician can do a full defibulation under anaesthesia which will not only remove the obstruction from the urinary flow but will also make intercourse much easier. She explained that the healing will probably take two weeks during which time Salha will take a course of antibiotics to clear the cystitis. **She was careful to explain that the defibulation is not a reconstruction** and that any further enhancement to the sexual relationship is not a matter of surgery but will **depend on how the couple will communicate with each other**. She referred her to the clinic counselor for more exploration of her concerns and expectations of the defibulation.

During the defibulation the physician noticed that the **clitoris was only partially removed** and was careful not to injure the sensitive tissue. Salha's wound healed uneventfully and the NP followed her up with monthly visits for six months to monitor changes in her menstrual symptoms. She performed several tests to exclude long term effects of urinary obstruction on the kidneys. She also performed high vaginal swabs and ultrasounds to check on the status of the uterus, tubes and ovaries.

Salha also continued to see the clinic counselor who helped her deal with relationship issues that emerged in the first year of her marriage. The NP continued to follow up her emotional and physical well being through three monthly visits. Both professionals learned that, although they cannot give Salha back her genitals or solve all her future problems, they can help her lead a satisfactory and normal life by providing trusted and caring support and services when she needs them.

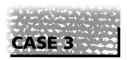

CASE 3

Hala is a 30 year old Egyptian housewife and mother

of a 3 year old daughter. She reported to the women's health clinic at her local public hospital with **severe vulval pain in the past 6 months which gets worse on intercourse**. On further questioning by the clinic's nurse she explained that she would like to have another child and was worried because **she has not succeeded in getting pregnant** for the last 2 years even though she has not used any contraception.

The nurse decided to **take her to a private room** and take a more detailed history. Her history revealed that she is married to her childhood sweetheart who has been working as a night shift taxi driver for the past 18 months. She reported that lately she has been having dreams in which she is being physically violated or her daughter is being forcibly circumcised. The nurse asked her if she was circumcised and she responded positively. She did not know what type of circumcision she had but she did remember all the details of the events even though she was eight years old when it occurred and she had not thought about it or remembered it all these years. She did not remember having any physical complications after the operation in fact she remembered being able to go back to school one week after the circumcision. The recent **flashes of memory and unpleasant dreams** started shortly after she attended a lecture at the local community center on the harmful effects of circumcision. She has also seen some programs on American television where they called it genital mutilation.

The nurse referred her to the fertility clinic after detailed recording of her history. On examination she was found to have **Type I FC/FGM** with a scar over the clitoral area 4 mm long. On careful examination with a blunt point she experienced **severe pain over the area of the scar**. There were no visible signs of inflammation in the vulva. Her pelvic examination showed normal sized anteverted uterus and normal sized ovaries.

The specialist started the first line of **tests for secondary infertility** including a sperm count and motility, a pap smear, high vaginal swab and a hysterosalpingogram. All were within normal limits. She also met with the couple and asked further about their sexual history. It soon became clear that because of the husband's night shifts and the wife's recent emotional difficulties and pain during intercourse they were having sex infrequently. The specialist explained the possibility of a **trapped clitoral nerve in the clitoral scar** as a cause for the pain during intercourse and that she will attempt to correct it with surgery but that there are no guarantees that it will work. She advised the couple to find more relaxed time to be alone to talk and relax into having sex and to do it more at the time of ovulation by using a special ovulation detection kit. The specialist performed a minor operation under general anaesthesia where she identified a thickened area of the scar. The scar was excised and the area buried in an inverted layer of mucosa. During the follow-up visits **the physician asked the couple if they intended to circumcise their daughter**. They both replied with a definitive no; they explained that now that they are better informed about the harms of female circumcision and have experienced its effect on their sexual relationship they are convinced it is not a good thing. They also added that there has been a group of them forming at the community center who are trying to encourage other families to abandon this practice and they have the support of their local religious leader.

Four weeks later Hala and her husband decided to go for a three months visit to their families in Egypt. Hala confided her troubles to her older sister who assured her that she too had periods of finding sex difficult in the past and advised her to go on a second honeymoon with her husband and offered to take care of the daughter. Hala and her husband spent two weeks alone in a seaside resort in Alexandria. Shortly after they returned to the U.S. Hala discovered that she was pregnant.

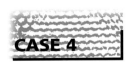

CASE 4

Amina is 19 year old Somali refugee woman who has been in the U.S. for 5 months only. **She was brought to the hospital in labor** accompanied by her husband and her sister in law. The two women did not speak English and the husband spoke enough for very basic communication. **She was a primigravida.** External examination of her vulval area revealed that **she had a long scar in place of her external genitals** with a posterior opening which allows the insertion of two fingers. Abdominal examination showed a pelvic presentation with the head engaged. She was experiencing contractions every fifteen minutes and foetal monitoring showed that the baby's heart beat was normal. She was taken to the delivery room and her husband requested that his sister stays with her during labor because he could not witness the delivery.

The senior resident was called to advise on the case. Upon examining the vulva he thought he remembered hearing about women who have ritual cutting of their genitals in some parts of Africa but he had never seen one before. He spoke to several midwives and one of them remembered that a colleague had worked in Somalia in the past. They managed to track her down where she was living in another state. Over the telephone they described to her what they saw and she explained that Amina was infibulated. She then explained that Amina needs to be defibulated in the second stage of labor just as the head is pushing to crown. She faxed them pages of **a book she had which shows how to perform defibulation** under local anaesthesia and how to stitch the edges afterwards.

The doctor tried to speak to the husband and to explain the procedure but **the language barrier was too great**. The husband gave the number of the local refugee resettlement agency and through them the hospital was able to get in touch with a Somali case worker who is fluent in English. The case worker attended the labor and facilitated the communication including the **signing of the consent form** and filling of various admission and payment forms. Amina had a healthy baby boy through an uneventful vaginal delivery within four hours of admission.

Two weeks later Amina came for her first post-partum follow up visit. She spoke to the nurse and physician through a women interpreter booked by the clinic through a local translation service. All was well with the baby but Amina was very concerned that **her infibulation site was left unstitched or "naked" as she expressed it**.

The senior resident presented Amina's case at the weekly departmental meeting. He had gathered medical information about defibulation and the legal status of re-infibulation in the U.S. After a rich discussion of the physical implications of re-infibulation as well as the psychological issues presented by Amina being uncomfortable with her genitals not infibulated, the hospital team decided on the following course of action:

1 Amina and her husband will be offered counseling to explain the effects of infibulation and to address their worries and concerns.

2 Amina will be put on a physical therapy regime of sitz baths and local wheat germ cream to help her accept the new feeling of her genitals.

3 If after adequate counseling and physical therapy Amina insists on re-infibulation the senior resident volunteered to do a partial infibulation that will not cover the urethra or vaginal opening free of charge.

After one month of physical therapy and weekly visits to the counselor Amina decided that she does not want to be re-infibulated. She has also been talking to other Somali women who delivered in the U.S. who encouraged her not to be re-infibulated. Her husband supported her decision.

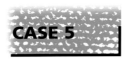

Awa is a 34 year old woman from Senegal who works as a hair braider and lives with her boyfriend and two teenage children. She came to the emergency room late one night with **sudden and excessive vaginal bleeding**. She gave a history of six weeks amenorrhea. Awa has been living in the U.S. for seven years and speaks enough English to express her self confidently.

On examination Awa had a bulky uterus with open os and moderate amount of bleeding and products of conceptions in the vaginal canal. She was diagnosed to have **a miscarriage in the sixth week of pregnancy**. She was admitted to hospital and scheduled for an emergency suction evacuation. During Awa's examination the attending nurse noticed that Awa had no clitoris and part of her labia minora was missing. She mentioned her observation to the examining physician who in his rush did not notice the look of the external genitals. During the evacuation procedure under general anaesthesia the physician confirmed the nurse's findings and documented the information in Awa's records.

Next morning Awa was due to be discharged from hospital and the physician came to see her before she left. After checking that she had no physical problems he asked her if she had planned to be pregnant and when she said that it was an unplanned pregnancy he asked if she wanted a referral to a family planning clinic. She said she always wanted to know about contraception but never found out where to go for information. He also mentioned that he noticed she was circumcised (he explained the findings and that her type of circumcision is referred to as type II) but does not believe that her circumcision should affect her recovery or any future pregnancy or delivery. Before leaving he gave her the address of the nearest Planned Parenthood clinic and invited her to ask any questions about the miscarriage and its possible consequences or about her circumcision. He also informed her that they have **social workers in the outpatient clinic** who can answer any questions she may have in the future.

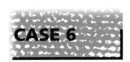

Yamisi Ajay is a **4 year old** Nigerian girl who was brought by her parents to the pediatric outpatient clinic **with fever for the past 24 hours**. On examination she was found to have a temperature of 101F and there was an area of **inflammation and tenderness in the vulva**. The pediatrician also noticed that **the clitoris and labia minora were missing** and replaced by an area of scar tissue on the inner side of the inflammation. She asked the parents what had happened to the genital area and they explained that she was circumcised when she was 2 years old back in Nigeria. The doctor was horrified at the thought and was not sure the parents were telling the truth. She had heard about female genital mutilation and that some immigrant families were having it done to their daughters in the U.S. She diagnosed the case as **cellulitis of the vulva**, admitted Yamisi to the pediatric ward, put the child on I.V. broad spectrum antibiotics and reported the case to the social worker for investigation.

The social worker interviewed the parents who both spoke good English. They reported that the father has been working in the U.S. for 8 years and visiting the family in Nigeria every year. The mother joined him with Yamisi and Peju, her 18 months old sister only six months ago. They repeated that Yamisi was circumcised back home when she was 2 years old and that after her circumcision she had a very bad infection and the wound did not heal for many weeks. They also said that they noticed the scar became red and hot several times but it had returned to normal again on its own.

When asked whether they intend to circumcise their 18 months old daughter the mother replied that she hopes to go visit her family the following year and that she is saving to have the ceremony done for Peju at that time. The social worker asked them to provide her with their passports and other documents to confirm their story that Yamisi has only been living in the U.S. for six months. Before their next meeting the social worker consulted a pamphlet she had in her files on the legal aspects of FC/FGM. **She called a legal advise center** listed in the pamphlet and spoke with one of the lawyers about the case she is investigating. The lawyer confirmed that if there is adequate evidence that the circumcision did not happen in the U.S., the social worker had no obligation to report it but if she was suspecting it did occur in the U.S. she should consider reporting it to the law enforcing agencies.

The Ajay family provided the required document in their next meeting with the social worker. Present at the meeting was a hospital lawyer who asked the family more questions and carefully examined the documents they provided. A committee made up of the social worker, lawyer, examining pediatrician and a hospital administrator met and after studying the evidence decided that they were satisfied that Yamisi was not circumcised in the U.S. and they will not report the case.

The social worker met with the parents again and **explained why they had to investigate the case**. She explained that FC/FGM is illegal in the U.S. and if they had done it here they would have been arrested and tried and if found guilty given a penalty of a fine, imprisonment or both and a criminal record. Also, depending on their immigration status they could also risk deportation.

She explained that the U.S. government has taken these legal measures to protect the health and welfare of children. She explained that although she understood that they did not mean to harm Yamisi by circumcising her she already suffered a lot from the procedure and could suffer more in the future. She strongly advised them not to circumcise Peju for her own sake. She too can have health problems. She added that the girls will grow up in America where other children are not circumcised and they will grow up feeling different and may get angry at their parents for cutting them.

Yamisi was discharged from hospital after two days with a continuing course of oral antibiotics. The social worker continued to see the family at their follow up outpatient visits and later by making home visits. She allowed them to ask many questions and responded sensitively to their concerns. She provided them with material produced by local community groups on the health, sexual and psychological effects of FC/FGM and the cultural and religious arguments why it should be stopped. She gave them the address of a local community group where they could go and talk to other African families opposed to the practice.

By the end of six months the social worker felt confident that the Ajay family will not circumcise their younger daughter and stopped visiting them. She hoped that her judgement in this case was right.

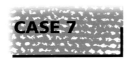

CASE 7

Aysha is a 17 year old high school pupil from Sierra Leone. She made an appointment to see the school nurse because her period was 6 days late. She has been having sex with her boyfriend for the past 3 months and she is not taking any contraception. The nurse advised her that it would be too early to detect a pregnancy and that she should wait for two weeks. If she is still not menstruating she will order her a pregnancy test.

She referred her to the guidance counselor who discussed with her whether she is really ready to be sexually active, or is she just responding to boyfriend and peer pressure. She also gave her **information on contraception, sexually transmitted disease and HIV/AIDS.** During the counseling Aysha mentioned her insecurity about not being attractive enough and **whether she will be "good enough" for the boys since she is circumcised.** Aysha remembered that she was circumcised at age 10 together with a group of other girls as part of their initiation ceremony into the secret society. She mentioned that her boyfriend is Caribbean and he does not know about her circumcision. She only talks about it with her sister who is also circumcised. She would never mention it to her American friends. She remembered that once there was a program on TV and some of her class mates asked her if she was mutilated and she denied it. She does not talk about it to her mother who speaks little English, and who does not understand her present reality in the U.S. She has mixed feelings about her identity and her culture. She is proud to be African and does not want to replace that with anything else. But sometimes she is not quite sure she belongs to Sierra Leonian culture. She **gets angry that she was circumcised but she knows that her parents did not mean to hurt her** and that they love her and her sister very much and have sacrificed a lot to give them the life they have in the U.S. She feels like she is living two separate lives. The one she shares with her

CASE STUDIES

family at home and the other which she has to adapt to in order that she is accepted in the American culture. She hopes to go back to her country one day and help her people but she does not know if she will fit. Her boyfriend understands many of the issues she is dealing with because he is from an immigrant family as well. That is why she feels she has to agree to having sex or she will loose him.

Aysha had her period three days after she visited the clinic. She was glad that she was not pregnant this time and promised herself that she will concentrate on her studies and deal with sex later.

FURTHER READINGS

Chapter 1

Lowry TP & Lowry TS. *The Clitoris*. St. Louis, MO, Warren H. Green Inc., 1976: 111–161.

Female Genital Mutilation. Report of a WHO Technical Working Group, Geneva, 17–19 July 1995. Geneva, World Health Organization, WHO/FRH/WHD/96.

Toubia N. & Izett S. *Female Genital Mutilation: An Overview*. Geneva, World Health Organization, 1998.

Chapter 2

Abdalla R. *Sisters in Affliction; Circumcision and Infibulation of Women in Africa*. London, Zed Press, 1982.

Assaad M. "A Harmful Practice Embedded in Culture and Tradition." *Report from the Seminar on Female Genital Mutilation*, Copenhagen, May 1995. Copenhagen, Ministry of Foreign Affairs/DANIDA, 1996.

Assad MB. "Female Circumcision in Egypt: Social Implications, Current Research and Prospects for Change." *Studies in Family Planning*. 1980, 11(1): 3–16.

Bashir L. "Female Genital Mutilation: Balancing Intolerance of Practice with Tolerance of Culture." *Journal of Women's Health*, 1997, 6 (1): 11–14.

Carr D. "Female Genital Cutting." *Findings from the Demographic & Health Surveys Program*, DHS 1997.

Dirie MA & Lindmark G. "Female Circumcision in Somalia and Women's Motives." *Acta Obstetrica et Gynecologica Scandinavica*, 1991, 50: 581–585.

Dorkenoo E. *Cutting the Rose: Female Genital Mutilation, the Practice and Its Prevention*. London, Minority Rights Publications, 1994.

El Dareer A. "Attitudes of Sudanese People to the Practice of Female Circumcision." *International Journal of Epidemiology*, 1983, 12: 138–144.

Eyega Z & Conneely E. "Facts and Fiction Regarding Female Circumcision/Female Genital Mutilation: A Pilot Study in New York City." *JAMWA*, Fall 1997, 52 (4): 174–78, 187.

Ghadially R. "Update on Female Genital Mutilation in India." *Women's Global Network for Reproductive Rights Newsletter*, January–March 1992.

Grisaru N, Lezer S, Belmaker RH. "Ritual Female Genital Surgery among Ethiopian Jews." *Archives of Sexual Behavior*, 1997, 26 (2): 211–215.

Kluge EH. "Female Circumcision: When Medical Ethics Confronts Cultural Value." *Canadian Medical Association Journal*, January 15, 1993, 148(2): 288–289.

Leonard L. "Female Circumcision in Southern Chad: Origins, Meaning and Current Practice." *Social Science and Medicine*, 1996, 43 (2): 255–63.

Saadawi N. *The Hidden Face of Eve*. London, Zed Press, 1977.

Toubia N. *Female Genital Mutilation: A Call for Global Action*, 2nd Ed. New York, RAINBQ, 1995.

Jones WK et al. "Female Genital Mutilation/Female Circumcision: Who is at Risk in the U.S.?" *Public Health Report*, 112, Number 5, September/October 1997.

Agugua NEN & Egwuatu VE. "Female Circumcision: Management of Urinary Complications." *Journal of Tropical Pediatrics*, 1982, 28: 242–252.

Aziz FA. "Gynecologic and Obstetric Complications of Female Circumcision." *International Journal of Gynecology and Obstetrics*, 1980, 17: 560–563.

Asuen MI. "Maternal Septicaemia and Death after Circumcision." *Tropical Doctor*, 1977, 7: 177–178.

DeSilvia S. "Obstetric Sequelae of Female Circumcision." *European Journal of Obsterics, Gynaecology and Reproductive Biology*, 1989, 32: 233–240.

Dirie MA & Lindmark G. "The Risk of Medical Complications after Female Circumcision." *East African Medical Journal*, 1992, 69:479–482.

Egwuatu VE & Agugua NEN. "Complications of Female Circumcision in Nigerian Igbos." *British Journal of Obstetrics and Gynaecology*, 1981, 88: 1090–1093.

Hathout HM. "Some Aspects of Female Circumcision with Case Report of Rare Complication." *Journal of Obstetrics and Gynaecology of British Empire*, 1963, 70: 505–507.

Horowitz CR & Jackson JC. "Female 'Circumcision: African Women Confront American Medicine." *JGIM*, August 1997, 12: 491–99.

McCaffrey M, Jankowska A, Gordon H. "Management of Female Genital Mutilation: The Northwick Park Hospital Experience." *British Journal of Obstetrics & Gynecology*, October 1995, 102(10): 787–90.

McCaffrey M. "Female Genital Mutilation: Consequences for Reproductive and Sexual Health." *British Association for Sexual and Marital Therapy*, 1995, 189–200.

Mustafa AZ. "Female Circumcision and Infibulation in the Sudan." *Journal of Obstetrics and Gynaecology of the British Commonwealth*, 1966, 73: 302–306.

Olamijulo SK et al. "Female Child Circumcision in Ilesha, Nigeria." *Clinical Pediatrics*, August 1983, 580–581.

Onuigbo WIB & Twomey D. "Primary Vaginal Stone Associated with Circumcision." *Obstetrics and Gynecology*, 1974, 44: 769–770.

Rushwan H. "Etiologic Factors in Pelvic Inflammatory Disease in Sudanese Women." *American Journal of Obstetric and Gyneocology*, 1980, 877–879.

Shandall AA. "Circumcision and Infibulation of Females: A General Consideration of the Problem and a Clinical Study of the Complications in Sudanese Woman." *Sudan Medical Journal*, 1967, 5: 178–212.

Shaw E. "Female Circumcision: Perception of Clients and Care Givers." *JACH*, April 1985, 33: 193–97.

Shorten A. "Female Circumcision: Understanding Special Needs." *Holistic Nursing Practice*, January 1995, (2): 66–73.

Stewart R. "Female Circumcision: Implication for North American Nurses." *Journal of Psychosocial Nursing & Mental Health Services*, April 1997, 35 (4): 35–8.

Woolard D & Richard E. "Female Circumcision: An Emerging Concern in College Health Care." *JACH*, March 1997, 45: 230–32.

World Health Organization, International Federation of Gynecology and Obstetrics. "Female Circumcision, Female Genital Mutilation." *International Journal of Gynecology and Obstetrics*, 1992, 37: 149.

Chapter 4

Baker C, Gilson G, Vill M & Curret L. "Female Circumcision: Obstetric Issues." *American Journal of Obstetrics and Gynecology*, 1995, 169 (6): 1616–18.

Daw E. "Female Circumcision and Infibulation Complicating Delivery." *The Practitioner*, 1970, 204:559–563.

McCleary P. "Female Genital Mutilation & Childbirth: A Case Report." *BIRTH*, December 1994, 21:4 221–23.

Newman M. "Safe Motherhood. Midwifery Care for Genitally Mutilated Women." *Modern Midwife*, June 1996, 6(6): 20–2.

Omer-Hashi K. "Female Genital Mutilation: Overview & Obstetrical Care." *The Canadian Journal of Obstetrics/Gynecology & Women's Health Care*, 1993, 5 (6): 538–42.

Chapter 5

Hedley R, Dorkenoo E. Child Protection and Female Genital Mutilation: *Advice for Health, Education and Social Work Professionals*. London, FORWARD Ltd., 1992.

Chapter 6

Guidance for Doctors Approached by Victims of Female Genital Mutilation, British Medical Association, January 1996.

Cross-Cultural Caring: A Handbook for Health Professionals in Western Canada. Edited by Waxler-Morison N, Anderson JM, Richardson E., Vancouver, University of British Columbia Press, 1990.

New York Task Force on Immigrant Health: Cross-cultural Care Giving in Maternal and Child Health: A Training Manual. New York, New York University School of Medicine, 1995.

Six Steps Towards Cultural Competence: How to Meet the Health Care Needs of Immigrants and Refugees. Recommendations from the Minnesota Public Health Task Force, Minnesota, Refugee Health Program, August 1996.

Chapter 8

Key F. "Female Circumcision/Female Genital Mutilation in the United States: Legislation & Its Implications for Health Providers." *JAMWA*, Fall 1997, 52 (4): 179–80, 187.

"Legislation on Female Genital Mutilation in the United States." *Reproductive Freedom in Focus*, The Center for Reproductive Law & Policy, Inc., October 1997.

UN Declaration on Elimination of Violence Against Women, December 1993, (United Nations General Assembly resolution 1386 (XIV)).

R

READINGS

APPENDICES

**TERMS USED FOR CIRCUMCISION
IN SOME OF THE COUNTRIES
WHERE IT IS PRACTICED**

Country	Language	Transliteration	Meaning
Burkina Faso	Bambara	Negekorosigui	Literally-when a woman goes under a knife. The term has political connotations and is not commonly used by the lay person.
		Kene-Kene	Circumcision/Excision
		Bolokoli	Literally-washing one's hands. It is unclear whether the term is used to imply that circumcision is cleanliness or that it refers to the circumciser washing hands after the cutting procedure.
Egypt	Arabic	Tahara	From the Arabic word "tahar" which means to clean or purify.
		Khitan	Circumcision (used for both male and female circumcision)
		Khifad	From the Arabic word "khafad" which means to lower. Refers to lowering of the height of the clitoris by cutting (rarely used in colloquial language)
Ethiopia	Amharic	Megrez	Circumcision/cutting
	Harrari	Absum	Name giving ritual
Eritrea	Tigregna	Mekhnishab	Circumcision/cutting
Gambia	Soussou	Lili	Cutting
Guinea	Malinké	Kileg/Digitongu	Ablution or cleansing. Both words are used inter-changeably to describe the practice.
Kenya	Kimeru	Gutanwa	The actual cutting in circumcision (used for both girls and boys) used by the Ameru ethnic group.
	Maa	Emorata	The actual cutting in circumcision (used for both girls and boys) used by the Maasai and Samburu ethnic groups who share the same language.
	Swahili (national language)	Kutairi (wasichana)	Kutairi literally means circumcision and is used for both girls and boys. When wasichana is added it becomes 'circumcision of girls.'
	Kikuyu	Kurua	To circumcise
	Kikuyu	Kuruithia airaetu	To circumcise girls
	Kikuyu	Irua	Ceremony

Country	Language	Transliteration	Meaning
Mali	Bambara	**Bolokoli**	Literally-washing one's hands. It is unclear whether the term is used to imply that circumcision is cleanliness or that it refers to the circumciser washing hands after the cutting procedure.
	Bambara	**Negekorosigui**	Literally-when a woman goes under a knife. The term has political connotations and is not commonly used by the lay person.
Nigeria	Igbo	**Ibi/Ugwu**	The act of cutting. It is used for circumcision of boys and girls (the Igbo language has several dialects. Other dialects within this language may have a different term for circumcision.)
Sierra Leone	Mandingo Soussou	**Sunna**	Sunna refers to a range of practices that follow the teachings of Islamic religion. This term is used by different groups of people of the Muslim faith in different countries to refer to female circumcision based on their understanding that the practice is recommended in the religion. The Soussou and Mandingo people are predominantly Muslim.
	Temeneè Mendeè Mandingo Limba	**Bondo**	An initiation/training which is an integral part of the passing onto adulthood. Those who participate in the training are considered initiated once they have been circumcised.
	Mendeè	**Sonde**	Same as Bondo
Somalia	Somali	**Gudiniin**	Circumcision (used for both girls and boys)
	Somali	**Halalays**	From the Arabic word "halal" which means 'sanctioned.' Used to imply purification or purity. Used mostly by the people of Northern Somalia or by Arabic speaking Somalis.
	Somali	**Qodiin**	Stitching, tightening or sewing. Used to refer to infibulation.
Sudan	Arabic	**Tahoor**	From the Arabic word "tahar" which means to clean or purify.
	Arabic	**Khifad**	From the Arabic word "khafad" which means to lower. Refers to lowering of the height of the clitoris by cutting (rarely used in colloquial language)

Appendix II UNITED STATES FEDERAL LEGISLATION ON FEMALE CIRCUMCISION/ FEMALE GENITAL MUTILATION.[1]

Legislation on FGM	Terms/Conditions
Statutory provision criminalizing the practice of FGM as part of the Illegal Immigration Reform and Immigrant Responsibility Act of 1996. Codified at 18 U.S. Code § 116.	It provides that "'whoever knowingly circumcises, excises, or infibulates the whole or any part of the labia majora or labia minora or clitoris of another person who has not attained the age of 18 years shall be fined under this title or imprisoned not more than 5 years, or both.'" The statute exempts a surgical operation if such operation is "'necessary to the health of the person on whom it is performed, and is performed by a person licensed in the place of its performance as a medical practitioner.'" The term "'health'" in this exemption is to be interpreted narrowly. The statute states that "'no account shall be taken of the effect on the person on whom the operation is to be performed of any belief on the part of that person, or any other person, that the operation is required as a matter of custom or ritual.'" The statute also excepts an operation if it is "'performed on a person in labor or who has just given birth and is performed for medical purposes connected with that labor or birth by a person licensed.... as a medical practitioner, midwife, or person in training to become such a practitioner or midwife.'"
Passed on September 30,1996 and entry into force on April 1, 1997.	

1. United States Federal Legislation on Female Circumcision/Female Genital Mutilation Source: "Legislation on Female Genital Mutilation in the United States." Reproductive Freedom in Focus, The Center for Reproductive Law & Policy, October 1997.

Appendix III **STATE LEGISLATION ON FEMALE CIRCUMCISION/ FEMALE GENITAL MUTILATION IN THE UNITED STATES[2]**

Legislation on FGM	Terms/Conditions
California The California Prohibition of Female Genital Mutilation Act. Criminal provisions in West's Annotated California Penal Code, § 273a. Passed in 1996 and entry into force on January 1, 1997.	The law amends the state penal code to provide that any person who violates a provision on child endangerment that prohibits any person from endangering a child to suffer physical, mental suffering, or injury by an act constituting "'female genital mutilation,'" "'shall be punished by an additional term of imprisonment in the state prison for one year.'" The penalty for endangering a child ranges from one to six years imprisonment.
Delaware Delaware Criminal Code, Delaware Code Annotated, title 11, § 780. Passed in 1996 and entry into force on July 3,1996.	FGM is classified as a class E felony, which is punishable by up to five years imprisonment. The law states that a person is guilty of FGM if he/she "'knowingly circumcises, excises or infibulates the whole or any part of the labia minora or clitoris of a female minor.'" In addition, a "'parent, guardian or other person legally responsible or charged with the custody of a female minor'" is also guilty of the same if he /she "'allows'" such acts to be performed on his/her daughter. A surgical procedure necessary to the "'health'" of a minor or which is "'performed on a minor who is in labor, or who has just given birth'" that is performed by a licensed physician, physician-in-training, or a licensed midwife is not considered FGM. A defense citing custom, ritual or standard practice or the consent of minor's parent or legal guardian is expressly disallowed.
Illinois Offense of FGM recently added to the Criminal Code of Illinois, Ill. Compiled Statutes, title 720, § 5/12-34. Entry into force on January 1,1998.	The offense is a class X felony, punishable by not less than six years or more than 30 years imprisonment. The law states that "'whoever knowingly circumcises, excises, or infibulates, in whole or in part, the labia majora, labia minora, or clitoris of another commits the offense of female genital mutilation.'" The statute prohibits the performance of FGM on any woman regardless of age. Consent to the procedure by a minor's parent or guardian is not a valid defense. Thus, it may be possible to argue that the consent of the

2. State Legislation on Female Circumcision/Female Genital Mutilation in the United States Source: "Legislation on Female Genital Mutilation in the United States." Reproductive Freedom in Focus, The Center for Reproductive Law & Policy, October 1997.

adult woman would be a sufficient defense. Exceptions to the prohibition are surgical procedures that are performed by a licensed physician for "'the health of the person'" or "'on a person who is in labor or who has just given birth and [are] performed for medical purposes connected with that labor or birth.'"

Maryland

An Act Concerning Health–Female Genital Mutilation, Annotated Code of Maryland, General Section 20-601 to 20-603

Signed by the Governor on April 28, 1998 and entry into force October 1, 1998.

FGM is considered a felony and carries a prison sentence not exceeding five years or a fine of not more than $5,000.00, or both. The law states that a person who "knowingly circumcises, excises, or infibulates the whole or any part of the labia minora or labia majora or clitoris of an individual who is under the age of 18 is guilty of female genital mutilation." A parent or legal guardian of an individual under 18 is also guilty of FGM if he or she knowingly consents to any of the procedures described above. Belief in custom or ritual cannot be used as a defense. The only exceptions to this law are instances where the procedure is "necessary to the health of the individual on whom it is performed" and for "medical purposes connected [with labor or giving birth]." In both cases the procedure may only be performed by a licensed medical professional.

Minnesota

Criminal code amended. See Minnesota Statutes,
§ 609.2245(1).

Passed in 1994.

The state amended its criminal code to declare that "'whoever knowingly circumcises, excises, or infibulates, in whole or in part, the labia majora, labia minora, or clitoris of another is guilty of a felony.'" Thus the statute prohibits the performance of FGM on anyone regardless of age. Consent to the procedure by a minor on whom it is performed or by the minor's parent is not a valid defense. It may be possible to argue that the consent of the adult woman would be a sufficient defense. Exceptions to this are surgical procedures performed by a licensed physician that are necessary for the health of a person, or that are performed for medical purposes on a person who is in labor or who has given birth.

New York

New York State Prohibition of Female Genital Mutilation Act. Criminal provisions in N.Y. Penal Law § 130.85.

Passed in September 1997 and entry into force in November 1997.

FGM is classified as a class E felony which is punishable by up to fours years imprisonment. The act states that a person is guilty of FGM when he/she "'knowingly circumcises, excises, or infibulates, the whole or any part of the labia majora, labia minora, or clitoris of another person who has not reached eighteen years of age.'" In addition, "'a parent, guardian or other person legally responsible and charged with the care and custody of a child less than eighteen years old, [who] knowingly consents to the circumcision, excision or infibulation of whole or part of such child's labia minora or labia majora or clitoris'" is guilty of FGM. Exceptions to this prohibition are when circumcision, excision or infibulation is "'necessary to the health of the person on whom it is performed, and is performed by a person licensed in the place of its performance as a medical practitioner.'" FGM is also permissible when it is "'performed on a person in labor or who has given birth and is performed for medical purposes connected with that labor or birth by a person licensed in the place it is performed as a medical practitioner or midwife.'"

North Dakota

A provision added to criminal code. See North Dakota Century Code § 121.1-36-01 (1995).

Passed on August 1, 1995.

FGM is classified as Class C felony which is punishable by up to five years imprisonment, a fine of $5,000 or both. The law states that "'any person who knowingly separates or surgically alters normal, healthy, functioning genital tissue of female minors is guilty of a class C felony.'" A surgical operation performed by a medical practitioner to correct "'an anatomical abnormality or to remove diseased tissue that is an immediate threat to the health of female minor'" does not violate this law, but beliefs about FGM that are based on custom, ritual, or standard practice may not be taken into consideration in determining liability.

Rhode Island

The Criminal Offenses Act of Rhode Island was amended to include a description of FGM in the definition of "'serious bodily injury.'" Rhode Island General Laws 11-5-2 (1996).

Passed in 1996.

Rhode Island's felony assault statute provides that where assault or battery, or both, result in "'serious bodily injury,'" the person committing such act "'shall be punished by imprisonment for not more than 20 years.'" "'Serious bodily injury means physical injury that....causes serious permanent disfigurement or circumcises, excises or infibulates the whole or any part of the labia majora or labia minora or clitoris of a person.'"

Tennessee

The Prohibition of Female Genital Mutilation Act of 1996. Tennessee Code Annotated § 39-13-110(a)(1996).

Entry into force on July 1, 1996

FGM is classified as a Class D felony and is punishable by not less than two years nor more than 12 years imprisonment and a fine not to exceed $5,000. This act states that "'whoever knowingly circumcises, excises or infibulates in whole or in part, the labia majora, labia minora or clitoris of another commits a Class D felony.'" Consent to the procedure "'by a minor or by the minor's parent'" cannot be used as a defense. Thus, it may be possible to argue that the consent of the adult woman would be a sufficient defense. Surgery that is performed by a licensed physician or physician-in-training and that is "'performed on a person in labor or who has given birth'" for medical purposes, is not violation of this law.

Wisconsin

Criminal code revision. Wisconsin Statutes § 146.35(1)(1995).

Passed on May 28, 1996.

The act prohibits the "'circumcision, excision or infibulation'" of the "'labia majora, labia minora or clitoris of female minor.'" The penalty for violating this act is a fine of up to $10,000 or five years in prison, or both. Exceptions are made for performing the procedure when it is "'performed by a physician ...and is necessary for the health of a female minor'" or is "'necessary to correct an anatomical abnormality.'" Neither consent by the female minor, or a parent of the minor, nor a custom or ritual requirements can be asserted as a defense.

> Note: Other States may be in the process of enacting legislations or may do so in the future. Please check your own state laws for the most recent status.

A

U.S. STATE LEGISLATION

APPENDIX III

African countries that have recently enacted specific laws criminalizing FC/FGM:	1996	Burkina Faso
	1994	Ghana
	1998	Ivory Coast
	1999	Senegal
	1998	Tanzania
	1998	Togo

Note: Most African countries have statutes in their criminal code against grievous bodily injury that can be invoked to prosecute those involved in FC/FGM.

African countries with governmental decrees:	Egypt (ministerial decree)

Non-African countries in which laws specifically criminalizing FC/FGM have been enacted:	1994	Australia First State Law enacted
	1997	Canada
	1994	New Zealand
	1996	Norway
	1982	Sweden
	1985	United Kingdom
	1997	United States Federal Legislation

Note: France is the only country that has prosecuted individuals for practicing FC/FGM, and it was done under existing child abuse laws.

The European Commission is currently considering the benefit of passing a unified European directive or regulation to pass specific laws against FC/FGM as opposed to relying on the existing child abuse laws.

Appendix V **FURTHER RESOURCES**

For information on local community groups and community education material contact:

RAINBQ
African Immigrant Program
915 Broadway, Suite 1109
New York, NY 10010
Tel: (212) 477-3318
Fax: (212) 477-4154
Email: rainbq@aol.com
http://www.rainbo.org

For legal information and questions contact:

Center for Reproductive Law
and Policy (CRLP)
International Program
120 Wall Street
New York, NY 10005
Tel: (212) 514-5534
Fax: (212) 514-5538
http://www.crlp.org

For further listing of published and unpublished literature on FC/FGM contact:

The FGM Resource Group
The Population Information Program
of the Johns Hopkins Center for
Communications Programs
POPLINE
111 Market Place, Suite 310
Baltimore, MD 21202-4012
USA
Tel: (410) 659-6300
Fax: (410) 659-6266
http://www.jhuccp.org

PLEASE NOTE:

RAINBQ has produced an illustrated quick reference guide outlining the most common types of FC/FGM and the steps of defibulation.

For further information or to order, contact RAINBQ.

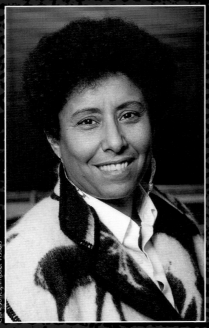

NAHID TOUBIA, M.D. was born in Khartoum, Sudan in 1951, and attended medical School in Egypt. In 1981 she became a fellow of the Royal College of Surgeons in England and the first woman surgeon in Sudan. She served as the head of the Pediatric Surgery Department at the Khartoum Teaching Hospital for many years. Recently, she worked for four years as an Associate for Women's Reproductive Health at the Population Council in New York City. She is currently an Adjunct Professor of Public Health at Columbia University School of Public Health and President of RAINBQ (Research, Action and Information Network for the Bodily Integrity of Women) in New York. She is also a member of several scientific and advisory committees of the World Health Organization, UNICEF and UNDP, and Vice-Chair of the Advisory Committee of the Women's Rights Watch Project of Human Rights Watch where she previously served on the Board of Directors. She publishes widely on issues of reproductive health, women's rights, and gender inequality particularly in Africa and the Middle East.

RAINBQ is an international, not-for-profit organization working on issues within the intersection of health and human rights of women. Starting with the issue of female circumcision/female genital mutilation (FC/FGM), RAINBQ explores means of preventing this and other forms of gender based violence. The organization's ultimate goal is to promote and protect women's reproductive and sexual health and rights.

RAINBQ provides technical assistance to international and donor agencies, and works in partnership with local organizations to develop and advance effective policies and programs to deal with these crucial issues. The organization's work is focused on programs in Africa and in African immigrant and refugee communities. The ██████████████████ are multi-cultural with a rich dive██████████████████ ces and personal backgrounds, a█████████████████.